MRCP (Paediatrics): Paediatric Picture Tests

MRCP (Paediatrics): Paediatric Picture Tests

Adam R. Craig

BSc (Hons), MB BS, MRCP (UK), MRCPCH
Tutor in Paediatrics
Department of Paediatrics and Child Health
St James's University Hospital, Leeds

Keith G. Brownlee

MB ChB, MRCP (UK), FRCPCH
Consultant Paediatrician
Department of Paediatrics and Child Health
St James's University Hospital, Leeds

W.B. Saunders Company Ltd

London • Philadelphia • Toronto • Sydney • Tokyo

W.B. Saunders   24–28 Oval Road
Company Ltd   London NW1 7DX, UK

The Curtis Center
Independence Square West
Philadelphia, PA 19106-3399, USA

Harcourt Brace & Company
55 Horner Avenue
Toronto, Ontario M8Z 4XS, Canada

Harcourt Brace & Company, Australia
30–52 Smidmore Street
Marrickville, NSW 2204, Australia

Harcourt Brace & Company, Japan
Ichibancho Central Building,
22-1 Ichibancho
Chiyoda-ku, Tokyo 102, Japan

© 1997 W.B. Saunders Company Ltd

A catalogue record for this book is available from the British Library

ISBN 0–7020–2163–6

Typeset by ColourZone, Isleworth, Middlesex
Printed and bound in Hong Kong by Dah Hua Printing Press Co. Ltd

Contents

Foreword

The aims of the MRCP (MRCPCH) Part 2 Examination are to assess the candidate's clinical knowledge, clinical judgement and ability to organise a management plan for the child. Although changes to the structure of the exam are likely within the next few years, neither the aims of the examination, nor the relevance of the information in this book, are likely to alter. The book will be helpful also for anyone wishing to learn more paediatrics, or who is preparing for clinical exams.

Many trainees are unsure about the examination syllabus. The most useful guide to the required standard, and the desired range of clinical knowledge, is in the 'Syllabus and Training Record for General Professional Training in Paediatrics', published by the Royal College of Paediatrics and Child Health 1996. It is worth remembering that there is differential marking for the questions in the written papers so that, for instance, a more important photographic subject has a maximum mark three times greater than a less important subject. Therefore, as is so for all medical practice, time given to learning about common and important problems, and those in which correct diagnosis can have an immediate impact on beneficial management, is more important that that devoted to rare and irremediable conditions.

Whether you are using this book to practice for the examination, or as a general aid to learning, don't waste it – don't cheat, don't look up the answers until you have thought carefully about the question and committed yourself to an answer; and if you want to make the most of it, write down your answer legibly and briefly, because that is what you have to do in an exam, and what you have to do in a child's medical records.

Sir Roy Meadow
Professor of Paediatrics & Child Health
St James's University Hospital
Leeds LS9 7TF   April 1997

Preface

The MRCP Part 2 examination is the final hurdle facing a paediatric SHO who wishes to become a specialist Registrar. Many candidates fail the examination because of poor preparation for the written paper. This book aims to help the reader acquire the two essential keys to success: examination technique and factual knowledge.

In Part One, we discuss the format of the written paper, concentrating on the photographic section. Advice is given on how to approach difficult questions and on ways of maximizing scores.

Part Two consists of six 20-question practice examinations, written in the membership style. To help the reader improve on their examination technique, we have included answer schemes that highlight the 'best' options. The questions are explained in detail with photograph descriptions, line drawings and revision notes. Up-to-date references are available for further reading.

By working through this book, we hope that the reader will be in a position for future success.

Adam Craig
Keith Brownlee

To our parents

Acknowledgements

We would like to thank Professor Sir Roy Meadow, Dr W. Ramsden, Dr S. Kinsey and Dr E. Kelly for kindly donating slides for this book, and Maria Khan of W.B. Saunders for her encouragement and support.

Part 1

How to Pass
the MRCP Part 2
Written Paper

The written paper consists of three sections: the grey cases, data inter-
pretation, and photographic material. Each section contributes an equal
number of marks to the final score. This book has been written to help
the candidate with the photographic section. However, many important
paediatric topics are summarized in short notes and these will be of value
when revising for all sections of the examination.

THE PHOTOGRAPHIC SECTION

You will be given 20 printed photographs or pairs of photographs, with a
separate question and answer booklet. You are allowed 50 minutes to
complete this section.

A wide range of images is used:

- Radiographs, CT scans, MRI scans, radioisotope studies, echocardio-
  grams.
- Patients with abnormal physical signs.
- Blood films, bone marrow aspirations and trephine biopsies.
- Microbiology slides and culture media.
- Microscopic and macroscopic pathology specimens.
- Urine/faecal samples.
- Normal patients.
- Retinal photographs.
- Others.

In general, abnormal physical signs and radiographs account for the
majority of images selected.

The questions are usually very short and may include an introductory
sentence giving details on the case. You may be asked for:

- A diagnosis/differential diagnosis.
- An associated sign, symptom or condition.
- An appropriate investigation.
- A treatment regimen.

3

ANSWERING QUESTIONS

Answers must be confined to the space provided. The examiners will disregard anything written outside this space, even if it is correct.

In theory each question should be allocated $2\frac{1}{2}$ minutes. However, some of the answers will be immediately apparent. Work through the paper quickly answering as many questions as possible, leaving out the difficult parts. You will then create extra time to complete the more taxing questions. Do remember to check that you have read each question correctly and that you have responded appropriately to each question.

Be methodical when analysing each photograph. For example, with a chest radiograph:

- Look at the labelling (left/right).
- Identify extraneous objects such as ECG leads.
- Look at the heart shadow and mediastinum.
- Look at the lung fields concentrating on the apices, the costophrenic and cardiophrenic angles, and the area behind the heart. Check for evidence of a pneumothorax.
- Look at the bony structures.
- Look at the soft tissues and abdomen
- Always compare the left-hand side of the image with the right-hand side.

Do try to be systematic so that under examination conditions you do not miss an obvious answer.

It is important to answer every question as the paper is NOT negatively marked.

Each question has a marking scheme with marks allocated for 'best' to 'worst' answers. The most *specific* and *complete* answer gains the most marks. For example, if asked for the diagnosis on a neonatal radiograph showing a left-sided diaphragmatic hernia, the best answer is 'left-sided congenital diaphragmatic hernia', not 'diaphragmatic hernia' which scores fewer marks. However, don't write waffle – the examiners hate it.

Use the full name of the condition. Think CONGENITAL/ ACQUIRED. Include the side of the lesion. Think RIGHT/LEFT.

If you cannot think of an answer to a question, the following suggestions should help you:

- Read the question carefully, looking for hints; it may be possible to answer the question using the written information alone.
- Are there subtle abnormalities that might give you clues to the

4

diagnosis? For example, an 'older' photograph may suggest a condition that is uncommon in modern practice.

- If you recognize the tissue, but not the abnormality, compose a list of possible conditions that may involve the tissue. Then try to exclude each possibility in turn. This technique could equally be applied to other photographs, such as pictures of abnormal hands or ears.

- If you are given a picture of something unusual that you do not recognize, try to think laterally. You are likely to be able to work out what it is. In past examinations, unusual pictures have included a meconium plug, redcurrant jelly stools and a stag horn calculus.

- Try to be as specific as possible. However, this does carry a risk. For example, you will not get any marks for incorrectly labelling acute lymphoblastic leukaemia as myeloid leukaemia, whereas a mark will be obtained for the answer 'acute leukaemia'.

- If you have no idea about a condition or syndrome, a non-specific answer may gain a mark; this may be the difference between a pass and a fail. For example, the identification of a child with Edward syndrome as a 'syndromic child' will probably score a mark.

- Play your hunches as they are often correct.

Don't forget that the image may be normal.

Finally, there is no substitute for a broad-based knowledge. By working through the 120 questions in Part Two, you will become familiar with many of the favourite examination topics.

Part 2

Where appropriate, we have included an answer scheme after each question. The first answer is the 'best' answer and would gain maximum marks. Thereafter, answers are ranked in descending order according to their suitability. Answers grouped together would gain an equal mark. Marking schemes have been avoided as they would be an unnecessary distraction to the reader.

Examination 1

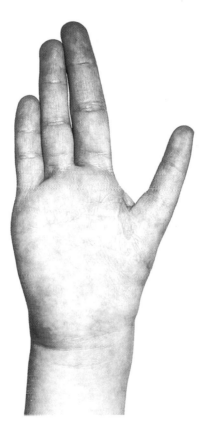

Questions

This 8 year old girl had multiple café au lait spots on her trunk.

(a) What procedure has been performed on her hand?

(b) What is the underlying diagnosis?

Answers

(a) Pollicization of the right index finger
      Surgical reconstruction of the right thumb
      Thumb reconstruction

(b) Fanconi's anaemia

Picture description

This child has three fingers and an apparent thumb. Pollicization of the right index finger has been performed and a scar is visible at the base of the reconstructed thumb.

Notes

- Fanconi's anaemia is a rare autosomal recessive disorder caused by the primary failure of stem cell production.
- Pancytopenia develops between 5 and 10 years of age.
- Associated features include skin pigmentation, café au lait spots, short stature, microcephaly, limb defects, renal abnormalities and genital hypoplasia.
- The bone marrow is hypocellular. HbF is increased (3–15%).
- The karyotype is normal, but there is excess *in vitro* chromosome fragility.
- The incidence of acute leukaemia and solid tumours is increased.
- The aplastic anaemia may respond to androgens (50%). Bone marrow transplantation has been successful.

Alter BP. Fanconi's anaemia and its variability. *British Journal of Haematology* 1993; **85**: 9–14.

Questions

(a) What is the diagnosis?

(b) List two conditions in which you would expect to find this abnormality?

Answers

(a) Coloboma of the left iris

(b) Trisomy 13
CHARGE syndrome
Goldenhar syndrome
Treacher Collins syndrome

Notes

- A coloboma is a developmental defect of the iris, and may involve the fundus and the optic nerve.
- Simple lesions can have an autosomal dominant pattern of inheritance.
- CHARGE syndrome: Coloboma, Heart defects, choanal Atresia, Retardation, Genital anomalies, Ears – deafness.

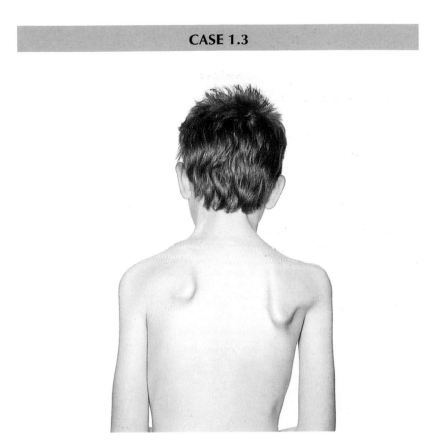

Questions

This 9 year old boy had facial weakness.

(a)   List two abnormalities.

(b)   What is the most likely diagnosis?

Answers

(a) Bilateral elevation and winging of the scapula
     Shoulder girdle muscle wasting

(b) Facioscapulohumeral muscular dystrophy

     Muscular dystrophy

Notes

- Facioscapulohumeral muscular dystrophy has an autosomal dominant inheritance with anticipation (subsequent generations develop a more severe illness, at an earlier age than the preceding generation).
- There is marked intrafamilial variability of phenotypic expression.
- The genetic defect is located on chromosome 4q.
- Symptoms of facial and shoulder girdle weakness usually present at the end of the first decade.
- The disease is progressive with successive involvement of the abdominal, foot extensor, upper arm and pelvic girdle muscles.
- Hearing loss and retinal vasculopathy are associated features, especially when the disease presents in early childhood.
- Calf hypertrophy is *not* a feature.

Brouwer OF, Padberg GW, Wijmenga C, Frants RR. Facioscapulohumeral muscular dystrophy in early childhood. *Archives of Neurology* 1994; **51**: 387–94.

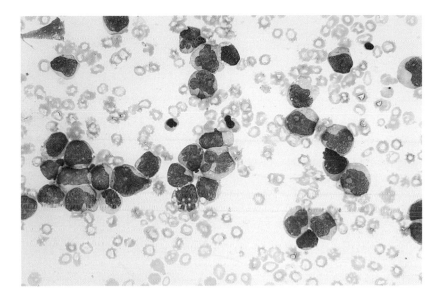

Question

This bone marrow aspirate is from a three year old girl.

What is the diagnosis?

Answers

Acute myeloblastic leukaemia

Acute leukaemia

Leukaemia

Picture description

The bone marrow is hypercellular with numerous myeloblasts. The myeloblasts are larger than red blood cells and have finely stippled nuclei with more than one nucleoli. Compared to lymphoblasts, they contain more cytoplasm and are more pleomorphic.

The appearance of the red blood cells is an artefact.

Notes

- Acute myeloblastic leukaemia (AML) comprises 20% of all childhood leukaemias.
- It is more common in older children and occurs equally in both sexes.
- Bloom's syndrome and Fanconi's anaemia predispose to AML.
- AML is classified according to morphology (M0 to M7).
- Gum hypertrophy is seen in the monocytic types (M4 and M5) and disseminated intravascular coagulation in type M3.
- The outlook is less favourable than for acute lymphoblastic leukaemia despite the use of intensive chemotherapy and bone marrow transplantation. The 5 year survival rate is 40%.

Ching-Hon P. Childhood leukemias. *New England Journal of Medicine* 1995; **332**: 1618–30.

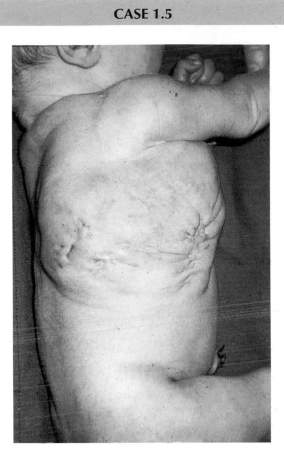

Question

What is the diagnosis?

Answers

Cystic hygroma
Lymphangioma
Haemangioma

Picture description

There is an irregular, lobulated mass arising from the right chest wall and axilla.

Notes

- A cystic hygroma is a developmental anomaly of the lymphatic system characterized by the formation of a multilocular cystic mass.
- Fifty per cent are present at birth, 80% detected before 2 years of age.
- Most occur in the head and neck, but they may develop in the mediastinum, axilla and chest wall.
- Examination reveals a soft, lobulated compressible mass that transilluminates brightly.
- Sudden enlargement may occur following haemorrhage or infection.
- Surgical excision is often difficult and has a significant morbidity and mortality.

Editorial. Cystic hygroma. *Lancet* 1990; **335**: 511–12.

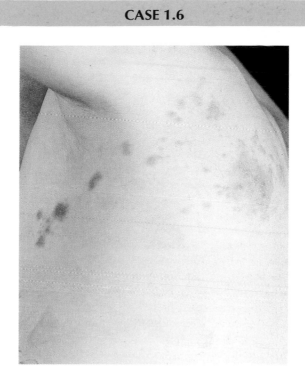

Question

What is the diagnosis?

Answers

Herpes zoster
Shingles

Notes

- Following chickenpox, the varicella zoster virus persists in a latent form within the dorsal root ganglia. It may later reappear as a painful vesicular rash in the dermatomes of the affected nerves.
- Pain, tenderness, fever and malaise may precede the onset of the rash.
- There is an increased incidence of zoster in immunocompromised children.
- Virus isolated from vesicle fluid can be identified by electron microscopy and virus culture, and by using specific monoclonal antibodies.
- Secondary bacterial infection is the commonest complication.
- Treatment with acyclovir may be effective if started at the onset of the infection.

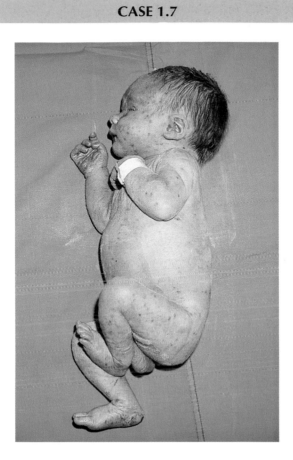

Questions

(a) Give three abnormalities in this newborn infant.

(b) What is the most likely diagnosis?

Answers

(a) Jaundice
    Purpuric rash
    Distended abdomen
    Wasted buttocks
    Post-mature skin

(b) Congenital infection/intrauterine infection
    Congenital toxoplasmosis
    Congenital cytomegalovirus infection
    Congenital rubella

    Congenital *Listeria* infection
    Disseminated intravascular coagulation secondary to sepsis
    Idiopathic thrombocytopenic purpura

    Leukaemia

Notes

Congenital toxoplasmosis
- The classical clinical triad is choroidoretinitis, hydrocephalus and diffuse intracranial calcification.
- Symptomatic infection is more likely when the infection occurs during the first trimester.
- Clinical features include rashes, jaundice, lymphadenopathy, hepatomegaly, splenomegaly and thrombocytopenia.
- Infected newborns can be treated with alternating courses of pyrimethamine/sulphadiazine and spiramycin until the age of 1 year.

Congenital cytomegalovirus (CMV) infection
- Between 0.5 and 1.5% of children are born with CMV infection.
- Over 95% of cases are asymptomatic.
- Infection during the first trimester poses the greatest risk of severe fetal damage.
- Clinical features include growth retardation, hypotonia, poor feeding, hepatosplenomegaly, seizures and microcephaly.
- The diagnosis is confirmed by isolating CMV from the infant's urine, saliva or cerebrospinal fluid.
- Periventricular calcification may be seen on skull radiograph.
- There is no evidence that antiviral agents alter the course of the disease.

Boppana SB, Pass RF, Britt WJ, Stagno S, Alford CA. Symptomatic congenital cytomegalovirus infection: neonatal mortality and morbidity. *Pediatric Infectious Disease Journal* 1992; **11**: 93–9.

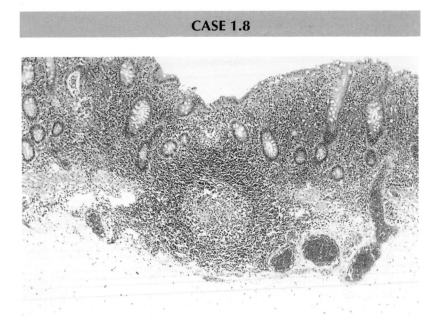

Question

This is a small bowel biopsy.

What is the diagnosis?

Answer

Crohn's disease

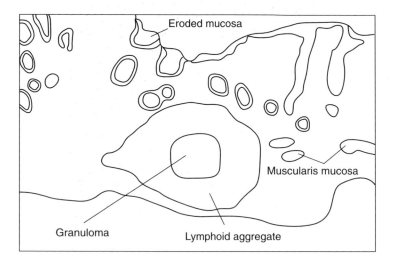

Picture description

There is superficial mucosal ulceration, together with haemorrhage within the lamina propria, and a lymphocytic infiltration extending through all the layers of the bowel wall. A large submucosal lymphoid aggregate surrounds a granuloma (a collection of epithelioid cells and multinucleated giant cells).

Notes

- In Crohn's disease, the inflammation extends through all layers of the bowel (transmural).
- Only 50% of cases show the typical granuloma; its absence does not exclude the diagnosis.
- Ulcerative colitis is essentially a disease of the mucosa, with a diffuse inflammatory infiltrate in the lamina propria, crypt abscesses and goblet cell depletion.

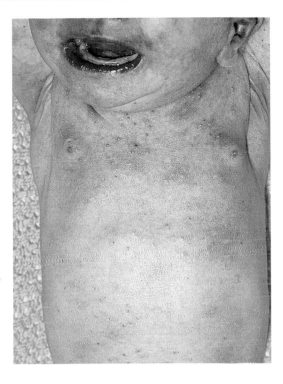

Question

What is the diagnosis?

Answer

Erythema toxicum neonatorum

Picture description

There are widespread pustules with surrounding erythema on the trunk of this newborn baby.

Notes

- Erythema toxicum is a benign, self-limiting eruption of unknown aetiology.
- It occurs in up to 50% of term infants.
- The lesions are rarely present at birth but appear within 72 hours, fading after several days.
- No therapy is indicated.

Question

This child presented with a vesicular rash involving his hands and feet. What is the most likely diagnosis?

Answers

Hand, foot and mouth disease
Herpes simplex

Notes

- Hand, foot and mouth disease is caused by enteroviruses, including coxsackie viruses A5 and A16.
- It occurs sporadically and in epidemics, especially in preschool children.
- The incidence is greater during the summer and autumn.
- Transmission is by droplet spread and the faecal–oral route.
- Incubation period 3–5 days.
- The illness starts as a mild pyrexia and malaise followed by a rash 3–5 days later.
- Lesions in the mouth begin as vesicles but rapidly erode into ulcers.
- Vesicles are more common on the dorsal surfaces of the hands and feet than on the palms and soles.
- The rash lasts about 1 week. The disease is self-limiting and requires only symptomatic treatment.

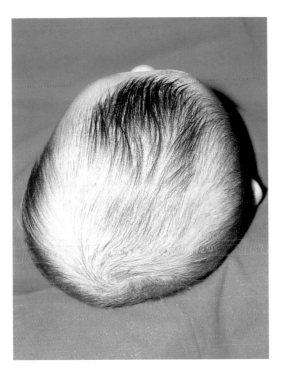

Question

What is the diagnosis?

Answers

Plagiocephaly
Skull asymmetry

Picture description

There is marked asymmetry of this infant's skull, with a prominent left occiput.

Notes

- Plagiocephaly (asymmetrical skull) is common in early infancy. The sutures are usually normal and the asymmetry resolves as the child grows.
- Rarely plagiocephaly results from the unilateral fusion of the coronal or lambdoid sutures. Corrective surgery performed during the first year of life is highly successful.
- Infantile idiopathic scoliosis is associated with plagiocephaly.

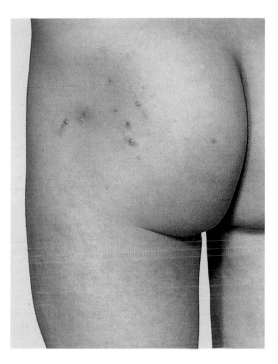

Question

What is the itchy rash of this child's buttock?

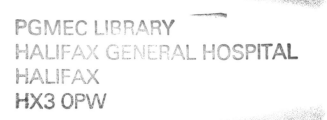

Answer

Molluscum contagiosum

Picture description

There are multiple pink-coloured papules overlying the left buttock.

Notes

- Molluscum contagiosum is a self-limiting cutaneous infection caused by a DNA virus of the poxvirus group.
- It commonly occurs in school-age children.
- Transmission is by direct contact with an infected individual or contaminant objects.
- The characteristic lesion is 2–5 mm across, a shiny papule with central umbilication.
- Crops usually appear on the trunk, neck and face.
- The condition may be exacerbated by the use of topical steroids.
- Most individual lesions regress within 2 months; the whole infection usually clears within 6–9 months.
- Treatment is not usually indicated.

Highet AS. Molluscum contagiosum. *Archives of Disease in Childhood* 1992; **67**: 1248–9.

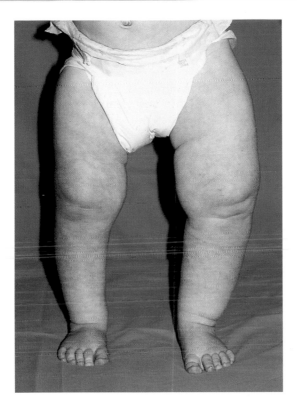

Questions

This child has a large birth mark on his face.

(a) What is the most likely diagnosis?

(b) List three alternative diagnoses.

Answers

(a) Klippel–Trenaunay–Weber syndrome

(b) Beckwith–Wiedemann syndrome
   Russell–Silver syndrome
   WAGR syndrome (Wilms' tumour, Aniridia, Genitourinary anomalies, Retardation)

   Tumour of left leg
   Deep vein thrombosis

Picture description

There is a generalized swelling of the left leg. This child had an underlying haemangioma as part of the Klippel–Trenaunay–Weber syndrome.

Notes

- Klippel–Trenaunay–Weber syndrome is a rare condition defined as the triad of a macular vascular naevus, skeletal overgrowth with soft tissue hypertrophy, and venous varicosities.
- The naevus is present at birth and usually involves a lower limb, but may involve the face or trunk.
- Pain, limb swelling and cellulitis may develop.
- Cardiac failure and thrombophlebitis are infrequent complications.
- Graduated compression bandages are used for the varicosities.
- Leg-length differences should be treated with orthotic devices to prevent the development of scoliosis. Large differences may need corrective surgery.

Samuel M, Spitz L. Klippel–Trenaunay syndrome: clinical features, complications and management in children. *British Journal of Surgery* 1994; **82**: 757–61.

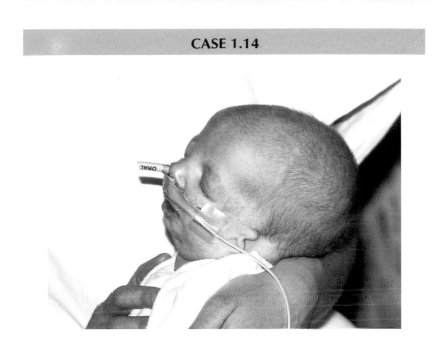

Question

What is the diagnosis?

Answers

Treacher Collins syndrome

Goldenhar syndrome

Picture description

The child's airway is being maintained by a nasopharyngeal tube. A naso-gastric tube is *in situ*. Dysmorphic features include a deformed pinna, an absent external auditory meatus, micrognathia, a downward sloping palpebral fissure and an abnormal hairline extending to the cheek.

Notes

- Treacher Collins syndrome (mandibulofacial dysostosis) is an auto-somal dominant disorder with variable expression, characterized by maldevelopment of the eyes, ears and mandible.
- Clinical features include coloboma, cleft palate, conductive deafness and congenital heart disease.
- Intelligence is usually normal.

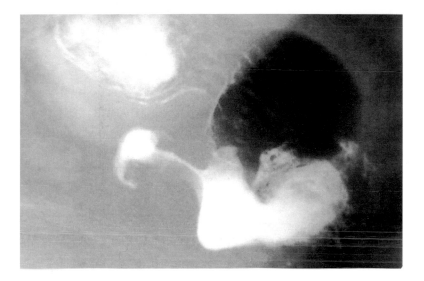

Question

This 4 week old boy was vomiting.

What is the diagnosis?

Answers

Congenital hypertrophic pyloric stenosis

Pyloric stenosis

Bowel obstruction

Malrotation
Duodenal atresia

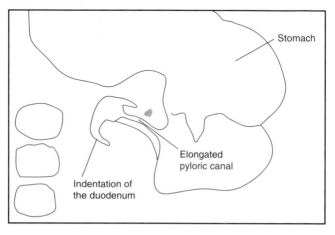

Picture description

This contrast meal examination revealed a narrowed and elongated pyloric canal (the 'string sign').

Notes

- Congenital hypertrophic pyloric stenosis occurs in about 1 in 400 live Caucasian births. Male:female ratio 4:1.
- Presents with vomiting, which is often projectile, in the third to fourth week of life. Infants are hungry to feed after vomiting.
- During a test feed, an olive-sized mass may be palpable in the right upper quadrant.
- Ultrasonography has replaced the contrast meal as the investigation of choice. The stenosed pylorus has a 'target' appearance.
- Two-thirds of patients will have a hypochloraemic metabolic alkalosis.
- Ramstedt's pyloromyotomy is the treatment of choice. Some centres are now performing laparoscopic pyloromyotomy.

Davenport M. ABC of general surgery in children. Surgically correctable causes of vomiting in infancy. *British Medical Journal* 1995; **312**: 236–9.

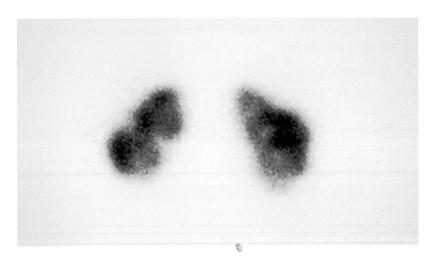

Questions

This investigation was performed on a 4 year old child, six months after a urinary tract infection.

(a) What is the investigation?

(b) What is the most likely cause for this appearance?

Answers

(a) ^{99m}Tc dimercaptosuccinic acid (DMSA) scan

Radioisotope scan

(b) Bilateral renal scarring secondary to vesicoureteric reflux
Vesicoureteric reflux

Acute infection
Pyelonephritis

Picture description

The kidney images have irregulars outlines with multiple defects in the uptake of isotope.

Notes

- DMSA is taken up by the proximal tubules and provides a functional assessment of the renal parenchyma.
- Renal scarring is suggested by persistent defects in isotope uptake.
- Temporary defects can be found following an acute urinary tract infection.
- Risk factors for developing renal scarring include vesicoureteric reflux (VUR), urinary tract obstruction, delayed treatment of infection and age less than 5 years.
- VUR is found in 30% of children investigated for urinary tract infection.
- Renal scarring is a major cause of hypertension and end-stage renal failure.

Question

This child walked with a limp.

What is the diagnosis?

Answers

Bilateral development dysplasia of the hips

Hip dislocation

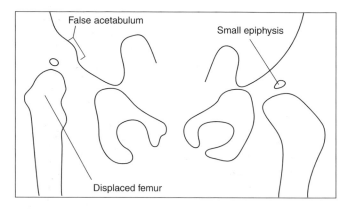

Picture description

Both hips are dislocated, the right more extensively. The ossification nuclei of the femoral heads are small and displaced laterally and superiorly. On the right side, a false acetabulum has formed with a shallow and underdeveloped true acetabulum.

Notes

- The term development dysplasia of the hip (DDH) refers to a wide spectrum of abnormalities ranging from capsular laxity to irreducible dislocation. Incidence 1 in 1000 live births.
- The cause is multifactorial. Predisposing factors include female sex (M:F ratio 1:9), breech presentation and positive family history.
- Physical examination may reveal limited hip abduction, leg shortening and additional thigh skin creases on the affected side, especially in the older child.
- In infants under 6 months of age, ultrasonography is now used in place of plain radiography as it is better at visualizing non-ossified tissues.
- If the diagnosis is missed at birth, children may present with delayed walking or an abnormal gait.
- The main objective of treatment is to achieve and maintain hip reduction so that the hip can resume normal development. Splinting, traction and open reduction are used according to the age of the child and the degree of hip abnormality.
- Children diagnosed after 6 months of age have a poorer outcome and a higher incidence of premature osteoarthritis.

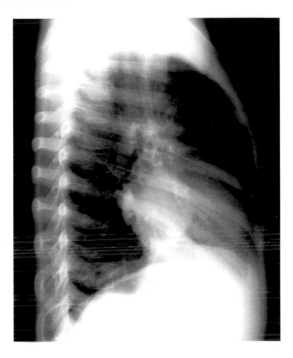

Question

This 8 year old girl presented with recurrent chest infections.

What is the most likely underlying diagnosis?

Answers

Bronchogenic cyst

Airway compression by enlarged lymph nodes
Staphylococcal pneumonia
Foreign body aspiration

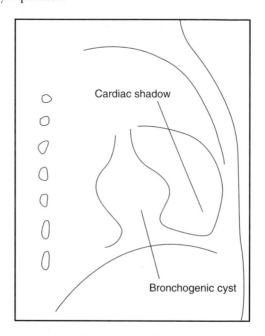

Picture description

There is a rounded opacity within the mediastinum.

Notes

- Bronchogenic cysts are derived from abnormal budding of the embryonic tracheobronchial tree.
- They are classified as central/mediastinal or peripheral/pulmonary.
- In general, they are single, unilocular and spherical in shape.
- They represent 10% of mediastinal masses in children.
- One-fifth are symptomatic. Clinical features include wheeze, stridor, recurrent pneumonia (secondary to airway compression) and obstructive emphysema.
- Cysts are well demonstrated using computed tomography (CT scanning) with contrast enhancement.

- The differential diagnosis is:
  - (i) Enlarged lymph nodes secondary to infection or neoplasm.
  - (ii) Pericardial cyst.
  - (iii) Oesophageal duplication.
  - (iv) Haemangioma.
  - (v) Lipoma.
- Even in the asymptomatic patient, surgical excision is indicated to prevent late complications (airway obstruction, infection and malignancy).

Kravitz RM. Congenital malformations of the lung. *Pediatric Clinics of North America* 1994; **41**: 453–72.

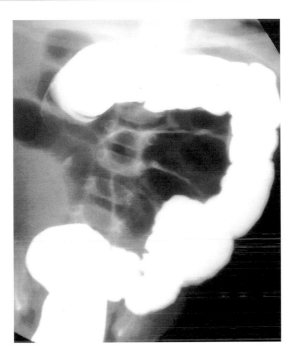

Question

This 3 month old boy was lethargic.

What is the most likely diagnosis?

Answers

Intussusception

Bowel obstruction

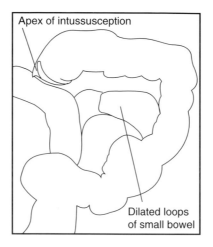

Apex of intussusception

Dilated loops of small bowel

Picture description

In this enema, the head of contrast has reached the apex of the intussusceptum. Small amounts of barium have passed between it and the wall of the intussuscipiens. The small bowel is dilated.

Notes

- Intussusception is the invagination of one bowel segment into an adjacent segment.
- The commonest site is ileocolic (80%).
- Incidence 1–2 per 1000 live births, peaking between 5 and 9 months.
- In the majority of cases no cause is found. However, intussusception does occur in association with viral illnesses, polyps, Meckel's diverticulum, Henoch–Schönlein purpura and lymphoma.
- Presenting features include paroxysmal crying, pallor, vomiting, and blood and mucus in the stools (redcurrant jelly).
- Abdominal palpation may reveal a tender sausage-shaped mass, usually at the hepatic flexure.
- Ultrasonographic examination of the mass reveals the characteristic 'target' appearance of the layers of intestine.
- Successful management depends on an early diagnosis, resuscitation and prompt reduction.

- Non-operative reduction, with air insufflation or a barium enema, should be attempted. The success rate with air insufflation is greater than 80%.
- Surgery is indicated in the presence of peritonitis and perforation, and if non-operative reduction fails.

Stringer MD, Pablot SM, Brereton RJ. Paediatric intussusception. *British Journal of Surgery* 1992; **79**: 867–76.

CASE 1.20

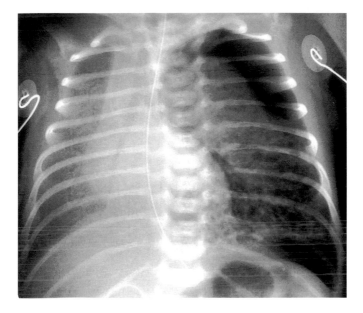

Questions

This ventilated preterm infant deteriorated suddenly.

(a)   List three abnormalities on this chest radiograph.

(b)   What immediate action would you take?

Answers

(a) Mediastinal shift to the right
Left-sided tension pneumothorax
Ground glass appearance of the right lung field.
Inferior displacement of the left hemidiaphragm

(b) Needle aspiration of left chest
Insertion of chest drain

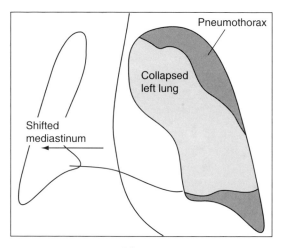

Notes

- In the neonatal period, pneumothorax is a complication of hyaline membrane disease, meconium aspiration syndrome or congenital lung malformation.
- In ventilated infants, the incidence of air leakage is increased by high peak pressures, prolonged inspiratory times and active expiration against the ventilator.
- Neonatal pneumothoraces may be asymptomatic or associated with severe respiratory distress and circulatory collapse.
- The risk of a pneumothorax can be reduced by using minimal ventilator pressures, faster ventilator rates and sedation/paralysis.
- The incidence of pneumothorax has declined since the introduction of exogenous surfactant.

Examination 2

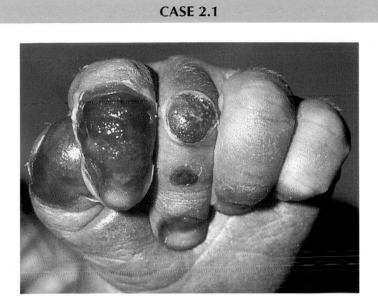

Questions

(a)   What is the most likely diagnosis?

(b)   List one differential diagnosis.

Answers

(a)   Epidermolysis bullosa

(b)   Scalded skin syndrome
      Burn
      Scald
      Non-accidental injury

Picture description

There are multiple skin erosions on the fingers that represent ruptured bullae. The nails are dysplastic.

Notes

- Epidermolysis bullosa is a group of conditions characterized by skin fragility with the formation of blisters at sites of pressure or trauma.
- The three categories are based on the level at which blistering occurs:
    (i)   Simplex – within the basal layer.
    (ii)   Junctional – epidermal–dermal junction.
    (iii) Dystrophic – within the dermis.
- Presentation is usually during the neonatal period.
- The mouth, gastrointestinal tract and trachea may become involved.
- Severe forms lead to scarring and contractures.
- Management involves topical and systemic antibiotics, wound compresses with non-adhesive dressings, protection of friction sites and nutritional support.

Eichenfield LF, Honig PJ. Blistering disorders in childhood. *Pediatric Clinics of North America* 1991; **38**: 959–76.

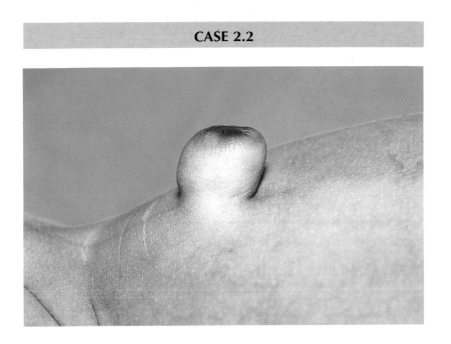

Question

What is the diagnosis?

Answers

Umbilical hernia

Paraumbilical hernia

Exomphalos

Notes

- An umbilical hernia results from a defect in the abdominal wall at the insertion of the umbilicus, with herniation of bowel into the redundant umbilical skin.
- Higher incidence in girls.
- Associated with Beckwith–Wiedemann syndrome, Hurler's syndrome, trisomy 18 and trisomy 13.
- Complications are very rare.
- Eighty per cent resolve by 4 years of age.
- Elective surgical repair is warranted if the hernia is symptomatic, or if it is still present as the child approaches school age (4–5 years).

Questions

(a) Describe two dysmorphic features,

(b) What is the most likely diagnosis?

Answers

(a)   Low-set ears
Micrognathia
Small chin
Short palpebral fissures

(b)   Edward syndrome
Trisomy 18

Chromosomal abnormality
Patau syndrome
Trisomy 13

Picture description

In addition to the features listed above the nasal alae are asymmetrical, suggesting the presence of a cleft palate.

Notes

- Edward syndrome has an incidence of 1 in 3000–5000 live births.
- Chromosome analysis shows a trisomy, mosaicism or an unbalanced translocation involving chromosome 18.
- Characteristic features include hypotonicity, cleft lip and palate, prominent occiput, widespaced nipples, overlapping fingers, cryptorchidism and rockerbottom feet.
- Cardiac and renal anomalies are common.
- Life expectancy is short with 90% dying within 3 months of birth.
- Babies who survive beyond infancy have severe disabilities.

Editorial. Clinical management of trisomy 18. *Lancet* 1992; **339**: 904.

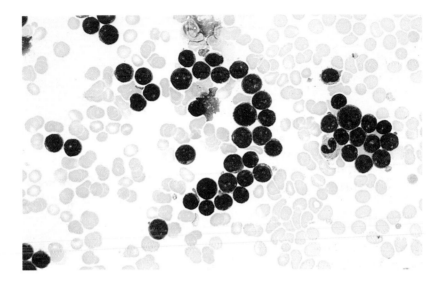

Question

This is a bone marrow aspirate.

What is the diagnosis?

CASE 2.4

Answers

Acute lymphoblastic leukaemia

Acute leukaemia

Leukaemia

Picture description

The bone marrow is hypercellular with numerous lymphoblasts. The lymphoblasts are larger than red blood cells, uniform in shape, have scanty cytoplasm and prominent nucleoli. Compared with myeloblasts, they contain less cytoplasm and are more uniform in shape.

The 'smudge' cell in the centre of the field is an artefact.

Notes

- Acute lymphoblastic leukaemia (ALL) accounts for 80% of all childhood leukaemias.
- The incidence is higher in trisomy 21, Bloom's syndrome and ataxia telangiectasia.
- Classification is according to morphology (French–American–British classification L_1, L_2, L_3) or immunophenotype (pre B-cell, B-cell, pre T-cell, T-cell, c-ALL, null).
- Overall 5 year survival rate is >70%.
- Poor prognostic factors include a white count >50 $\times$ 10^9 at presentation, central nervous system disease, mediastinal mass, male sex, age <2 years, age >10 years, B-ALL and the Philadelphia chromosome.

Ching-Hon P. Childhood leukemias. *New England Journal of Medicine* 1995; **332**: 1618–30.

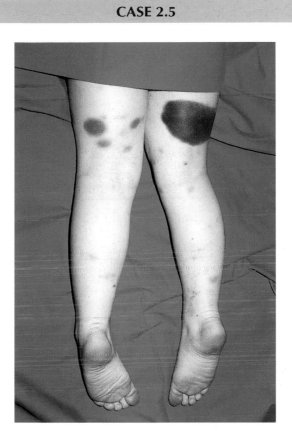

Question

What is the diagnosis?

Answers

Multiple congenital melanocytic naevi
Multiple congenital pigmented naevi

Multiple naevi
Pigmented naevi

Picture description

There are multiple brown pigmented lesions of varying sizes on the thighs and legs.

Notes

- Multiple congenital pigmented naevi are present at birth and increase in number over the first year of life.
- Lesions may be verrucose, nodular or flat, brown, blue or black, and hairy or hairless.
- Naevi over the head and neck may be associated with leptomeningeal melanocytosis.
- Congenital giant naevi (>20 cm in diameter) occur in 1 in 20000 newborns and often have a 'garment' distribution on the trunk and limbs. The risk of malignant transformation during childhood is high and early excision is recommended.

Rhodes AR. Important melanocytic lesions in childhood and adolescence. *Pediatric Clinics of North America* 1991; **38**: 791–809.

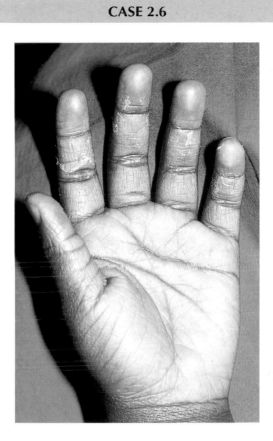

Question

What is the most likely diagnosis?

Answers

Kawasaki disease
Mucocutaneous lymph node syndrome

Picture description

The skin on the fingers and palm is peeling.

Notes

- Kawasaki disease is an acute, febrile, mucocutaneous syndrome of unknown aetiology.
- It commonly occurs in children under 4 years of age.
- The diagnosis can be made in the presence of a fever persisting for at least 5 days, plus four of the following criteria:
  (i)   Eyes – bilateral conjunctivitis.
  (ii) Lymph nodes – cervical lymphadenopathy.
  (iii) Skin – polymorphous exanthema.
  (iv) Hands and feet – reddening, oedema, desquamation.
  (v)   Mouth – mucositis, reddening, strawberry tongue.
- Other finding include anaemia, leucocytosis, thrombocytosis and a raised ESR.
- The differential diagnosis includes measles, scarlet fever, staphylococcal 'scalded skin' syndrome, drug reactions and juvenile chronic arthritis.
- Treatment is with aspirin and immunoglobulins.
- If untreated, 20–25% of patients develop coronary artery abnormalities (dilatation, aneurysms).
- Death is usually a result of cardiac complications. With treatment the mortality rate is less than 1%.

Kawasaki T. Kawasaki disease. *Acta Paediatrica* 1995; **84**: 713–15.

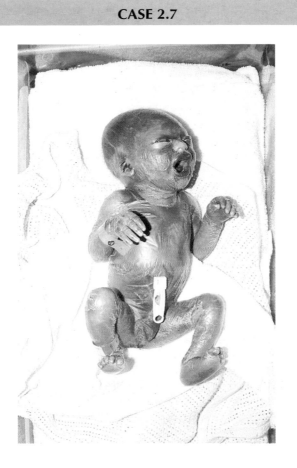

Question

What is the diagnosis?

Answers

Collodion baby
Congenital ichthyosis

Picture description

This newborn infant has bilateral ectropion and is covered by a shiny, thick, taut membrane. The mouth is fixed in a circular shape.

Notes

- A collodion baby is usually the presenting feature of one of the congenital ichthyoses, most often the lamellar variety.
- Occasionally there is normal skin beneath the collodion membrane.
- Hair may be absent or protrude through the covering.
- Desquamation of the membrane begins shortly after birth, and is complete in 10–14 days.
- Complications include infection, hypothermia and hypernatraemic dehydration from excessive transdermal fluid loss.

Shwayder T, Ott F. All about ichthyosis. *Pediatric Clinics of North America* 1991; **38**: 835–57.

Questions

(a) List three abnormalities on this small bowel biopsy.

(b) What is the most likely diagnosis?

Answers

(a) Absent villi
Hypertrophied crypts
Increased lymphocytic infiltration within the epithelium and lamina propria

(b) Coeliac disease
Gluten-sensitive enteropathy

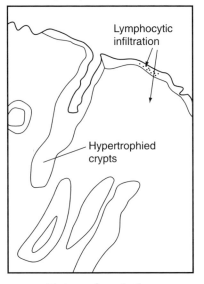

Picture description

This jejunal biopsy shows the typical features of subtotal villous atrophy.

Notes

- Coeliac disease is a disease of the small bowel characterized by an abnormal small intestinal mucosa, associated with intolerance to gluten.
- The incidence is 1 in 2000 in the United Kingdom and 1 in 300 in Ireland.
- The pathogenesis is believed to be a combination of cereal toxicity, genetic disposition and environmental factors.
- Ten per cent of patients have a first-degree relative with the condition.
- Presentation is usually during infancy or early childhood with diarrhoea, vomiting and failure to thrive.
- Removal of gluten from the diet leads to a full clinical and histological remission. Re-exposure to dietary gluten results in recurrence of the intestinal mucosal abnormality in 95% of individuals.

- Serum IgA antigliadin, IgA antireticulin and IgA antiendomysium antibodies are valuable in both the diagnosis and monitoring of cases.
- Strict adherence to a gluten-free diet is recommended to avoid the late development of bowel lymphoma or carcinoma.

Littlewood JM. Coeliac disease in childhood. *Baillière's Clinical Gastroenterology* 1995; **9**: 295–327.

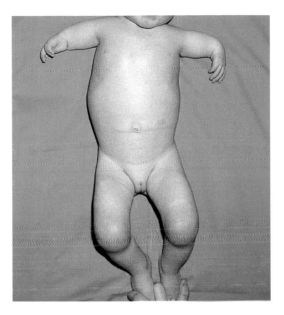

Question

This child has an atrial septal defect.

What is the most likely diagnosis?

Answers

Holt–Oram syndrome
VATER/VACTERL syndrome
Thrombocytopenia and absent radii (TAR) syndrome

Picture description

The upper limbs are poorly developed with dysplastic ulnae and absent radii.

Notes

- Holt–Oram syndrome (hand–heart syndrome) is an autosomal dominant condition with variable penetrance. The main features are upper limb defects (thumb and radial hypoplasia) and cardiovascular defects (atrial and ventricular septal defects).
- VATER/VACTERL syndrome: Vertebral anomalies, Anal atresia, Cardiac defects, Tracheo-oesophageal fistula, Radial and Renal dysplasia, Limb defects.

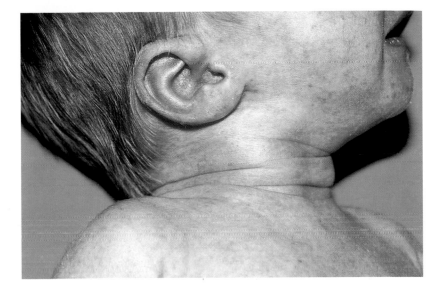

Question

This 4 week old baby was reported to be 'looking to the left'.

What is the diagnosis?

Answers

Right sternocleidomastoid tumour
Congenital muscular torticollis

Picture description

The baby's head is rotated with the occiput pointing towards the right shoulder. A swelling is visible within the middle portion of the right sternocleidomastoid muscle.

Notes

- Congenital muscular torticollis usually develops within 4–8 weeks of birth.
- Tumours are believed to result from injury to the muscle at birth.
- A non-tender, soft, mobile mass can be palpated overlying, or within, the sternocleidomastoid muscle.
- Treatment with passive stretching is usually effective in restoring neck movement.
- If the deformity persists after 1 year of age it is unlikely to resolve spontaneously. Surgical division of the sternocleidomastoid muscle, with or without lengthening, is indicated.

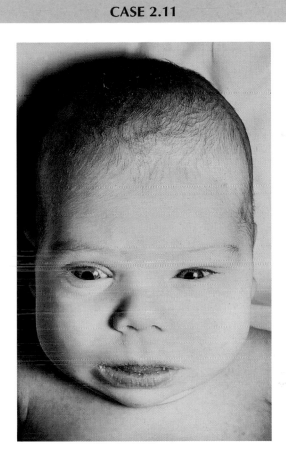

Question

What is the diagnosis?

Answer

Congenital hypothyroidism

Picture description

The baby has an expressionless face, puffy eyes, a hirsute forehead and a large tongue.

Notes

- In congenital hypothyroidism, the majority of affected infants have thyroid dysgenesis or agenesis. Dyshormonogenesis and transient hypothyroidism are rarer.
- The male to female ratio is 1:2.
- Early detection and treatment of congenital hypothyroidism is essential to avoid long-term sequelae.
- Most screening programmes measure thyroid stimulating hormone (TSH) concentrations and diagnose hypothyroidism on the basis of a raised TSH level. This method will not detect secondary hypothyroidism.
- Clinical features include prolonged physiological jaundice, feeding difficulties, somnolence, hypothermia and constipation.
- Noisy breathing and apnoeic episodes may result from upper airway obstruction secondary to macroglossia.
- Untreated, there is gradual progression to physical and mental retardation.
- In the majority of cases, thyroxine replacement results in normal growth and intelligence. However, some studies have reported lower intelligence in infants with very low pretreatment thyroxine levels, despite early treatment.

Grant DB. Congenital hypothyroidism: optimal management in the light of 15 years' experience of screening. *Archives of Disease in Childhood* 1995; **72**: 85–9.

Question

This child refused to weight bear on her left leg.

What is the most likely diagnosis?

Answer

Septic arthritis

Picture description

The left ankle is swollen and inflamed.

Notes

- In septic arthritis the joint may be invaded via a penetrating wound, by blood spread or from an adjacent osteomyelitis.
- *Staphylococcus aureus* is the commonest pathogen. Prior to the introduction of the Hib vaccination programme, *Haemophilus influenzae* type B was the commonest pathogen.
- Neonatal septic arthritis is caused by *Staphylococcus aureus*, group B streptococci, *Escherichia coli* or *Candida albicans*.
- In sexually active teenagers, gonococcal infection can cause both monoarticular and polyarticular sepsis.
- Septic arthritis should be treated quickly to prevent permanent damage to the articular cartilage.
- Management: antibiotics, irrigation and drainage, and immobilization of the joint in a functional position.
- Long-term problems: reduced limb growth, early degenerative changes and limited joint movement.

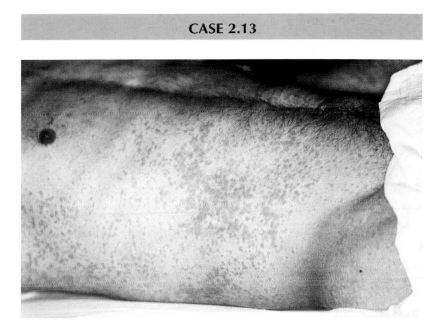

Question

This 14 year old boy was treated by his family doctor for a sore throat.

What is the most likely underlying diagnosis?

Answers

Infectious mononucleosis
Glandular fever
Epstein–Barr virus infection

Drug hypersensitivity

Picture description

There is a widespread erythematous maculopapular rash on the trunk and back.

Notes

- The commonest presenting feature of infectious mononucleosis is a sore throat (often with cervical lymphadenopathy).
- It is usually caused by the Epstein–Barr virus (EBV), but cytomegalovirus (CMV) and *Toxoplasma gondii* infections can cause a clinically indistinguishable syndrome.
- Antibiotics, in particular ampicillin, can precipitate a generalized hypersensitivity rash during an EBV or CMV infection.

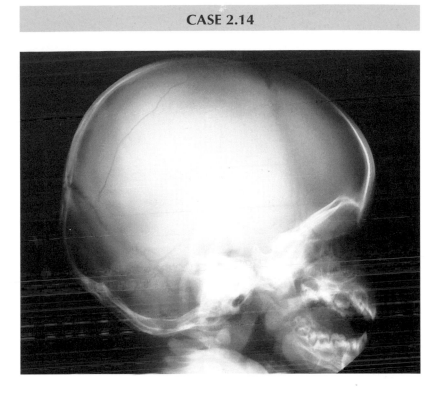

Question

What is the abnormality on this lateral skull radiograph?

Answers

Parietal skull fracture
Skull fracture

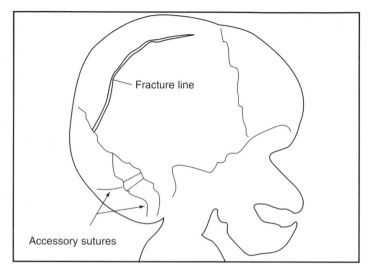

Picture description

A linear lucency is visible within the parietal bones. Multiple accessory sutures within the occipital bone are normal variants.

Notes

- Fractures of the skull can be easily confused with vascular markings or normal variants, such as a metopic suture (between two halves of the frontal bone) or an intraparietal suture.
- Fractures are sharply demarcated, straight and translucent lines with parallel margins.
- Vascular markings are less translucent, not sharply demarcated, symmetrical, and have a branching pattern.
- Depressed fractures appear as lines of increased density.

Nicholson DA, Driscoll PA, Hodgkinson DW, St C Forbes W. Skull. In: Nicholson DA, Driscoll PA, eds. *ABC of Emergency Radiology*. London: BMJ Publishing Group, 1995: 72–8.

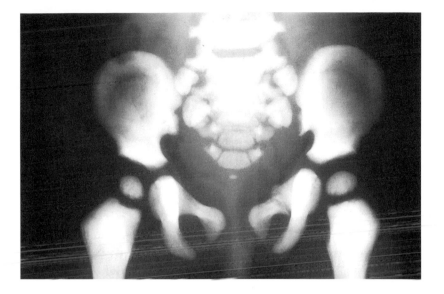

Questions

(a) List two abnormalities.

(b) What is the most likely diagnosis?

Answers

(a)   Dense bone with absent corticomedullary differentiation
      Transverse fracture of the left superior pubic ramus

(b)   Autosomal recessive osteopetrosis
      Osteopetrosis

Notes

- Osteopetrosis is caused by defective bone resorption with a characteristic increase in bone density and skeletal bone mass.
- Incidence estimated at 1 in 200 000 live births.
- The autosomal dominant form leads to mild disease in adult life.
- The autosomal recessive form occurs in infancy and is more severe. Problems include cranial nerve entrapment, bone marrow failure and recurrent fractures. Most children die within the first decade of life.
- Allogeneic bone marrow transplantation is the only curative option.

Gerritsen EJA, Vossen JM, van Loo IH, Hermans J, Helfrich MH, Griscelli C, Fischer A. Autosomal recessive osteopetrosis: variability of findings at diagnosis and during the natural course. *Pediatrics* 1994; **93**: 247–53.

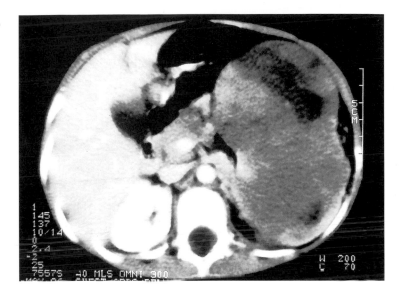

Question

This 5 year old girl presented with abdominal pain. A contrast-enhanced CT was performed.

What is the most likely diagnosis?

Answers

Left-sided Wilms' tumour

Neuroblastoma

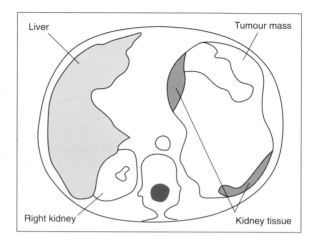

Picture description

There is a large mass, containing areas of fluid and necrosis, arising from the left kidney. A peripheral rim of normal kidney tissue is visible.

Notes

- Wilms' tumour is the commonest abdominal malignancy of childhood.
- Incidence 1 per 15 000 live births. Mean age at diagnosis 3.5 years.
- Bilateral tumours occur in approximately 5% of cases.
- Associated conditions include aniridia, hemihypertrophy, genitourinary abnormalities, neurofibromatosis and the Beckwith–Wiedemann syndrome.
- An 11q13 interstitial deletion is associated with Wilms' tumour and aniridia.
- Tumours commonly present as an asymptomatic abdominal mass or with abdominal pain (with or without haematuria).
- Successful treatment requires complete surgical excision, radiotherapy and chemotherapy depending on the stage of the disease.
- Overall 5 year survival 84%. With favourable histology survival is 90–95%.

Caty MG, Shamberger RC. Abdominal tumors in infancy and childhood. *Pediatric Clinics of North America* 1993; **40**: 1253–71.

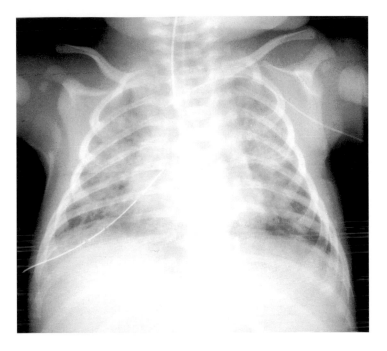

Question

This term infant developed respiratory distress shortly after birth. The Apgar score was 5 at 1 minute and 6 at 5 minutes.

What is the diagnosis?

Answers

Meconium aspiration syndrome

Aspiration pneumonia
Congenital pneumonia
Group B streptococcal pneumonia

Hyaline membrane disease

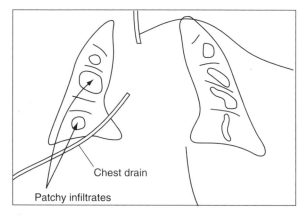

Chest drain

Patchy infiltrates

Picture description

The infant is intubated. Two chest drain are *in situ*. The lung fields are overinflated with widespread patchy infiltrates.

Notes

- Meconium stained liquor is found at about 10% of term deliveries, with an increased incidence in post-term and small-for-dates babies. Premature infants rarely pass meconium except in cases of congenital listeriosis.
- In meconium aspiration syndrome (MAS) the lungs are stiff and have reduced compliance. There is air trapping and marked ventilation–perfusion mismatching.
- Effective aspiration of meconium from the airways, both when the head crowns and immediately following delivery, significantly improves the outcome.
- MAS is managed with minimal handling, oxygen, intravenous fluids, antibiotics and mechanical ventilation.
- Complications include pneumothorax, pneumomediastinum and persistent fetal circulation.
- Deaths results from respiratory failure, persistent fetal circulation and air leaks.
- MAS predisposes to long-term respiratory disease in childhood.

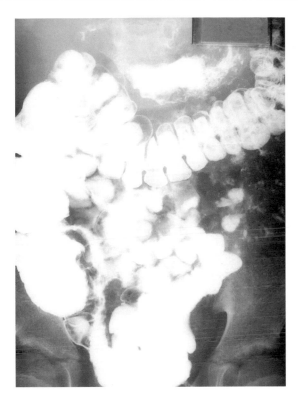

Question

What is the most likely diagnosis?

Answers

Crohn's disease

Inflammatory bowel disease

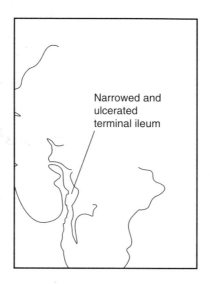

Narrowed and
ulcerated
terminal ileum

Picture description

In this double contrast barium enema, the terminal ileum is narrowed and ulcerated.

Notes

- In early Crohn's disease of the small bowel, contrast examination reveals aphthous ulceration and coarsening of the villous pattern. As the disease progresses, deep ulceration and inflammatory polyps develop. The mucosal pattern is eventually lost and the small bowel appears rigid.
- In Crohn's colitis, the earliest sign of disease on contrast examination is aphthous ulceration. With disease progression, the ulcers coalesce to form linear ulcers which may trap barium giving a striped appearance. Transmural ulceration appears as 'rose-thorn' or 'collar stud' ulcers. Colonic narrowing, cobblestoning, fistulae and sinuses develop later.

Caroline DF, Friedman AC. The radiology of inflammatory bowel disease. *Medical Clinics of North America* 1994; **78**: 1353–85.

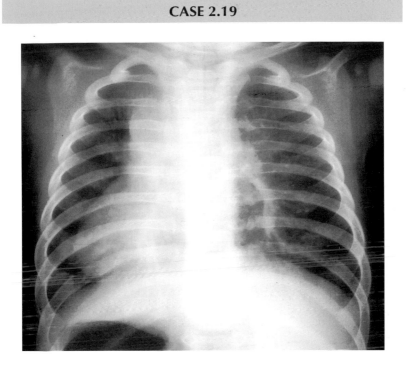

Questions

(a) Give two abnormalities on this chest radiograph.

(b) What is the most likely diagnosis?

Answers

(a)   Dextrocardia
  Situs inversus
  Absent left gastric bubble or right gastric bubble
  Bilateral bronchial wall thickening

(b)   Kartagener's syndrome
  Primary ciliary dyskinesia
  Primary ciliary dyskinesia with situs inversus viscerum

  Dextrocardia
  Situs inversus

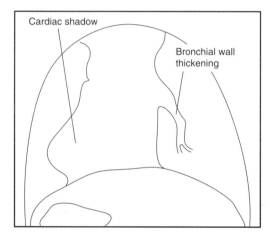

Notes

- Kartagener described the triad of bronchiectasis, sinusitis and situs inversus. The common abnormality is the absence or reduced number of dynein arms within the cilia.
- The term primary ciliary dyskinesia is now used as only 50% of patients with this abnormality have situs inversus.
- Clinical features include a chronic productive cough, chronic rhinitis, nasal polyposis, recurrent maxillary sinusitis, and recurrent otitis media.
- Bronchiectasis may develop in early childhood.
- Most men are sterile. Women may have reduced fertility.
- Nasal mucociliary clearance is prolonged. Nasal cilia may be obtained for analysis from inferior turbinate brushings.
- Abnormal motility is seen on light microscopy with the characteristic ultrastructural defect visible on electron microscopy.
- Irreversible lung damage is minimized by the early recognition and treatment of infections.

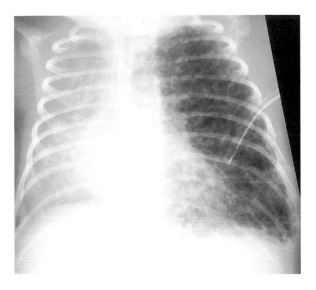

Question

What is the diagnosis?

Answer

Pulmonary interstitial emphysema

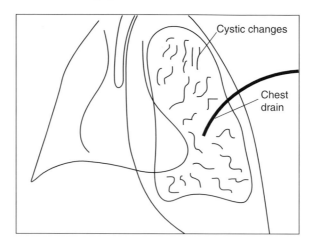

Picture description

An endotracheal tube (tip at the carina), nasogastric tube and left chest drain are *in situ*. The left lung field is overinflated, displacing the mediastinum to the right. It contains multiple, small, cystic radiolucencies with adjacent areas of alveolar collapse.

Notes

- Pulmonary interstitial emphysema (PIE) results from gas trapping within the perivascular bundles of the lungs.
- Lung perfusion and ventilation are disrupted resulting in hypoxaemia and carbon dioxide retention.
- Treatment options include conservative measures, selective intubation of the contralateral bronchus and high-frequency oscillatory ventilation.
- The incidence of bronchopulmonary dysplasia is increased following PIE.

Examination 3

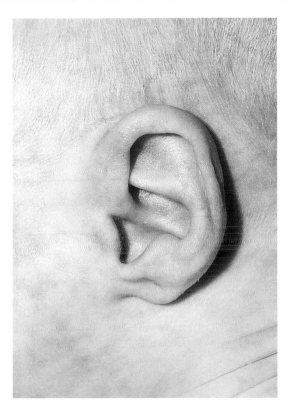

Question

What is the diagnosis?

Answer

Beckwith–Wiedemann syndrome

Picture description

There is a horizontal crease on the left ear lobe.

Notes

- Beckwith–Wiedemann syndrome (BWS) is characterized by macroglossia, gigantism, exomphalos, visceromegaly and hypoglycaemia.
- Incidence 1 in 14 000 live births.
- The BWS gene is situated at the 11q15.5 locus.
- Hypoglycaemia occurs in the majority of patients, but is usually mild and transient.
- Macroglossia may cause feeding difficulties, delayed speech and obstructive apnoea. Surgical reduction is performed in up to 50% of cases.
- Long-term problems include behavioural and learning difficulties.
- BWS predisposes to Wilms' tumour, adrenocortical carcinoma, hepatoblastoma and neuroblastoma, particularly in patients with a duplication of the 11p15 band.

Elliot M, Maher ER. Beckwith–Wiedemann syndrome. *Journal of Medical Genetics* 1994; **31**: 560–4.

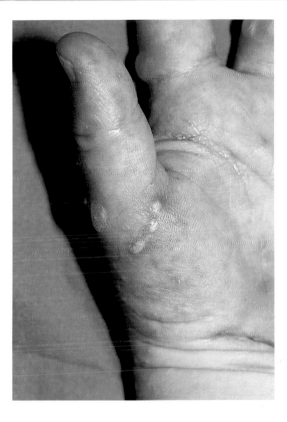

Questions

(a) List three abnormalities.

(b) What is the diagnosis?

Answers

(a) Pustules
     Vesicles
     Papules
     Linear burrows in finger webs

(b) Scabies

     Herpes simplex

Notes

- Scabies is a contagious infestation by the mite *Sarcoptes scabiei*.
- The female mite burrows into the keratin layer of the skin to lay eggs. On hatching they produce an intensely irritating eruption which is usually worse at night.
- The burrows are classically seen on wrists, palms and between the fingers.
- In children under 2 years the head and neck may be involved.
- Allergic reactions to the mite and its products are common, producing nodular and urticarial reactions.
- Secondary infection is common.
- The presence of burrows is almost diagnostic. Burrow scrapings identify ova and mites.
- All contacts and members of the patient's household should be treated simultaneously.
- Irritation may continue for up to 2 weeks after treatment. The papular lesions may persist for many months.

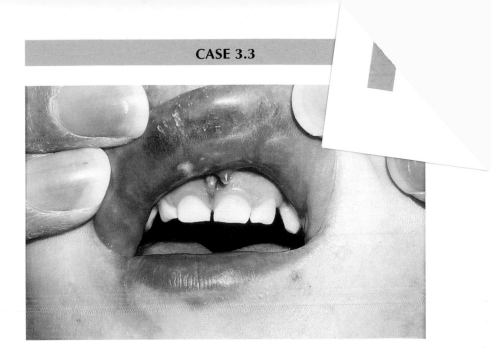

Question

List two abnormalities.

Answers

Torn upper/lingual frenulum
Aphthous ulcer

Scarred frenulum
Ruptured frenulum

Notes

- Injuries to the mouth are common in non-accidental injury and can be the result of rough feeding practices.
- Aphthous ulcers are common in children; the aetiology is unknown. They may be due to allergy or autoimmune conditions. Topical antibiotics and steroids can be beneficial.

Question

A 6 year old girl presented with pallor.

What is the most likely diagnosis?

Answers

Hereditary spherocytosis

Spherocytosis

Picture description

Spherocytes are densely staining cells that are smaller than normal red blood cells.

Notes

- Hereditary spherocytosis is the commonest haemolytic anaemia and results from a red cell membrane defect.
- Loss of the membrane causes the cells to form into rigid spheres which become trapped and then destroyed in the spleen.
- Prevalence 1 in 5000.
- Inheritance is usually autosomal dominant with variable expression.
- The main clinical features are mild jaundice, pallor and splenomegaly.
- There is often a positive family history of recurrent anaemia, gallstones or splenectomy.
- Osmotic fragility is increased.
- Severely anaemic patients and moderately anaemic but symptomatic patients undergo splenectomy. It is best avoided in early childhood because of the risk of severe infection.
- Pneumococcal vaccination should be administered prior to surgery with prophylactic penicillin V post-splenectomy.

Questions

This newborn baby was jaundiced.

(a)   What is the underlying diagnosis?

(b)   List three other abnormalities you would expect to find.

Answers

(a) Down syndrome

(b) Hypotonia
Microcephaly
Flattened occiput
Upward slanting eyes
Epicanthal folds
Protruding tongue
Clinodactyly of the fifth digit
Single palmar crease
Wide gap between the first and second toes

Picture description

The iris is speckled (Brushfield spots).

Notes

- Down syndrome has an incidence of 1 in 700 live births.
- The majority of cases are caused by trisomy 21 (95%), with the rest a result of translocations or mosaics.
- The risk of non-dysjunction causing trisomy 21 increases with maternal age. A woman between 40 and 44 years of age has a 20-fold increased risk compared with a woman aged between 20 and 24 years.
- Congenital heart disease is very common and responsible for one-third of deaths.
- Hypothyroidism occurs in 15% of cases.
- Chronic serous otitis media produces conductive hearing loss in up to 90% of children.
- There is a 1% lifetime risk of developing acute leukaemia. Chemotherapy remission rates are reduced.
- After the fourth decade, Alzheimer disease develops in approximately 15% of individuals.

Hayes A, Batshaw ML. Down syndrome. *Pediatric Clinics of North America* 1993: **40**: 523–35.

Newton RW, Newton JA. Management of Down's syndrome. In: David TJ, ed. *Recent Advances in Paediatrics*, Vol. 10. Edinburgh: Churchill Livingstone, 1992: 21–35.

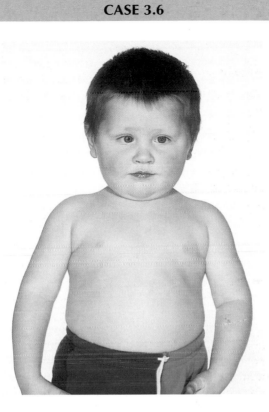

Questions

This boy suffered from recurrent wheeze.
A blood count revealed an eosinophilia.

(a) List two abnormalities.

(b) What is the overall diagnosis that explains both these abnormalities?

Answers

(a)   Harrison's sulcus
      Convergent right squint

(b)   Toxocariasis

Notes

- Toxocariasis is due to an infection by *Toxocara canis* and *Toxocara cati*, common gut parasites of dogs and cats respectively.
- Human disease is predominantly caused by *T. canis*, and mainly affects children aged 1–6 years.
- *Toxocara* eggs are ingested when a child eats contaminated soil, sand or vegetables.
- There are two distinct forms of the disease caused by larvae invading tissue:
    - (i)   Visceral larva migrans (VLM) results in fever, malaise, cough, bronchospasm, hepatomegaly and eosinophilia.
    - (ii) Ocular larva migrans (OLM) tends to occur in older children and is rarely accompanied by eosinophilia. The dead larva causes a granulomatous reaction in the retina. Presenting features include leucocoria, squint and impaired vision.
- VLM is diagnosed on the basis of the clinical picture accompanied by eosinophilia. Serum *Toxocara* antibodies are not reliable in the acute infection. Treatment is primarily symptomatic. Antihelminthics have limited success.
- OLM is diagnosed clinically from the appearance of the inflammatory mass in the retina. Antihelminthics are not effective, but topical or systemic steroids may be of benefit.
- Toxocariasis could be largely prevented if cats and dogs were regularly dewormed and prevented from defaecating in public places.

Kerr-Muir MG. *Toxocara canis* and human health. *British Medical Journal* 1994; **309**: 5–6.

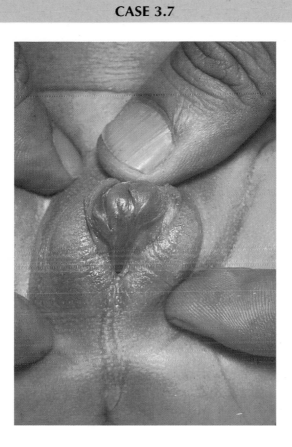

Questions

This 1 month old girl presented with vomiting.

(a) What is the most likely diagnosis?

(b) List one test that would confirm your diagnosis.

Answers

(a) Congenital adrenal hyperplasia
21-hydroxylase congenital adrenal hyperplasia
Adrenogenital syndrome

(b) Plasma 17-hydroxyprogesterone level

Adrenocorticotrophic hormone
Plasma renin
Plasma testosterone
Urinary steroid profile

Picture description

The genitalia are ambiguous with clitoromegaly and posterior fusion of the labia majora.

Notes

- Congenital adrenal hyperplasia (CAH) is a rare autosomal recessive condition with a partial or complete enzyme deficiency in cortisol and/or aldosterone synthesis.
- 21-hydroxylase deficiency accounts for 95% of cases and has an incidence of 1 in 14000 live births.
- The gene has been localized to the short arm of chromosome 6 close to the HLA locus.
- The classical disease occurs in two forms: simple virilizing and salt-losing.
- Salt-losing individuals are at risk of an adrenal crisis. Vomiting, diarrhoea, dehydration and circulatory collapse may develop during the neonatal period, requiring resuscitation with normal saline and hydrocortisone.
- Late-onset disease may present with adrenarche, virilization, hirsutism, menstrual abnormalities and infertility in females.
- Antenatal diagnosis during the first trimester is available.
- Long-term management: oral glucocorticoids and, if there is salt-loss, mineralocorticoid replacement.
- The degree of control of the condition can be monitored by measuring 17-hydroxyprogesterone and renin levels, together with growth and bone maturation.
- In some centres dexamethasone is used during early pregnancy to reduce virilization in affected females.

Czernichow P, Sizonenko PC. Paediatric endocrine and metabolic emergencies. In: Burger AG, Philippe J, ed. *Baillière's Clinical Endocrinology and Metabolism* 1992; **6**: 193–216.

Question

This rash failed to respond to treatment with topical steroid and antifungal agents.

What is the most likely diagnosis?

Answer

Psoriasis

Picture description

There is a pink scaling rash, with irregular margins, extending outside the nappy area.

Notes

- Psoriasis may present as a 'nappy rash'. Scaling is often limited because of the hydrating effects of the nappy.
- A positive family history can aid the diagnosis.
- The rash does not respond well to hydrocortisone/antifungal preparations. Tar preparations are more effective.
- Antifungal treatment is recommended as psoriasis can be precipitated by *Candida albicans*.

Mallory SB. Neonatal skin disorders. *Pediatric Clinics of North America* 1991; **38**: 745–61.

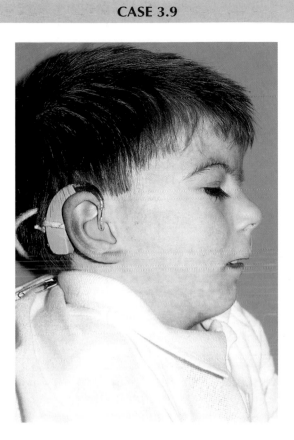

Question

What is the most likely diagnosis?

Answer

Cornelia de Lange syndrome

Picture description

This child is wearing a hearing aid, has long eyelashes, thin lips and prominent eyebrows that meet in the midline (synophrys).

Notes

- Cornelia de Lange syndrome is a sporadically occurring condition characterized by impaired growth, learning difficulties, microcephaly and hirsutism.
- Incidence is between 1 in 30 000 and 1 in 60 000 live births.
- Other features include intrauterine growth retardation, thin down-turned lips, low hair line, antimongoloid slant, low set ears and a broad nasal bridge.
- Hypoplasia of the feet and hands is common.
- One-third have major limb malformations, mainly involving the ulnar.
- Two-thirds die in the first year of life, predominantly as a result of pulmonary aspiration.

Jackson L, Line AD, Barr MA, Koch S. De Lange syndrome: a clinical review of 310 individuals. *American Journal of Medical Genetics* 1993; **47**: 940–6.

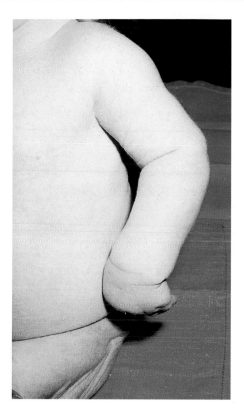

Question

What is the diagnosis?

Answer

Left Erb's palsy

Picture description

The left arm lies beside the trunk in the 'waiter's tip' position. It is internally rotated at the shoulder, extended at the elbow, with forearm pronation and wrist flexion.

Notes

- In Erb's palsy, roots C5–6 are damaged with denervation of the deltoid, supraspinatus, biceps and brachioradialis.
- Injuries are due to traction on the brachial plexus during delivery. In severe trauma the phrenic nerve may be involved with paralysis of the ipsilateral hemidiaphragm.
- Klumpke's palsy is rarer and results from damage to C8–T1. The clinical presentation is one of weakness of the wrist flexors and intrinsic muscles of the hand. Horner's syndrome may be present.
- Treatment: passive physiotherapy and splinting to avoid contractures.
- Ninety per cent of brachial plexus injuries recover within 6 months. A persistent deficit carries a poor prognosis. Neuroplasty may be beneficial.

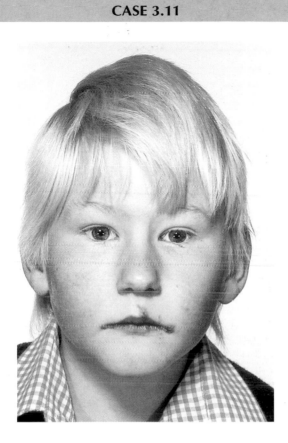

Question

This 9 year old child had feeding difficulties during the first six months of life.

What is the most likely diagnosis?

Answer

Prader–Willi syndrome

Picture description

This child has several features of Prader–Willi syndrome – fair hair, blue eyes, a narrow bifrontal diameter and a thin upper lip.

Notes

- Prader–Willi syndrome has an incidence of 1 in 10 000 births.
- Most cases are due to a deletion in the long arm of the *paternal* chromosome 15. Some cases are due to uniparental maternal disomy.
- Decreased fetal movements may be observed.
- In the newborn period, infants are hypotonic, have a weak cry and require tube feeding. Scrotal hypoplasia and cryptorchidism are common.
- During infancy and early childhood development is delayed, particularly speech and gross motor skills.
- Hyperphagia and behavioural problems make parenting difficult.
- Obesity begins at about 2 years of age. Strict dietary supervision is necessary to control food intake.
- The diagnosis is made on clinical grounds and by using molecular genetic techniques.

Donaldson MDC, Chu CE, Cooke A *et al.* The Prader–Willi syndrome. *Archives of Disease in Childhood* 1994; **70**: 58–63.

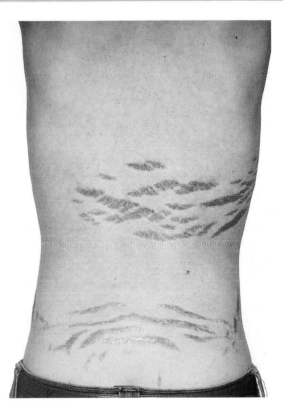

Questions

This 14 year old boy suffers from nephrotic syndrome.

(a)   Name this skin lesion?

(b)   How is it caused?

Answers

(a) Striae

(b) Corticosteroid therapy
     Prednisolone

Picture description

There are multiple red streaks of thin skin over the lower thoracic and lumbar regions.

Notes

- Long-term oral and topical steroids cause skin damage.
- The skin becomes thin and fragile, with spontaneous bruising, striae and telangiectasia.
- Thinning is reversible on withdrawal of the steroid. The striae and telangiectasia are permanent.

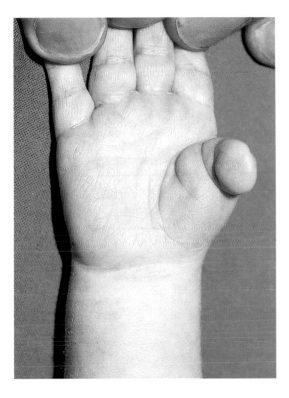

Question

What is the most likely diagnosis?

Answer

Rubinstein–Taybi syndrome

Picture description

The right thumb is broad and radially angulated.

Notes

- Rubinstein–Taybi syndrome results from a 16p13 – deletion.
- In infancy feeding and respiratory problems are common.
- Features: microcephaly, short stature, beaked nose, low-lying philtrum, cryptorchidism, broad toes and learning difficulties.
- The differential diagnosis of a broad thumb includes Apert, Carpenter and Larsen syndromes.

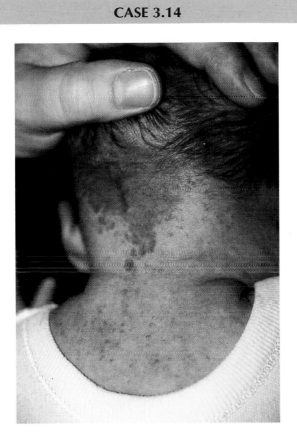

Question

What is the abnormality?

Answers

Capillary haemangioma
Stork mark

Cavernous haemangioma
Strawberry mark

Picture description

There is a pinkish flat lesion on the nape of this baby's neck.

Notes

- A capillary haemangioma is a well circumscribed defect of dermal capillaries found in up to 50% of babies on the nape of the neck, forehead and eyelids.
- Facial lesions usually fade over the first 2 years of life. Lesions on the nape may persist.

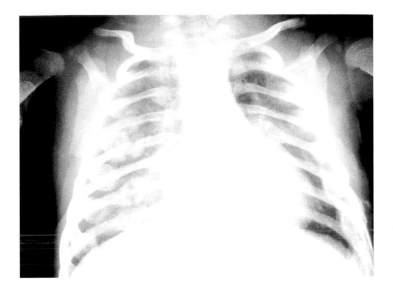

Question

What is the most likely cause for the abnormalities on this radiograph?

Answer

Non-accidental injury

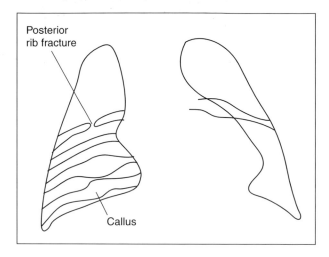

Posterior
rib fracture

Callus

Picture description

There are posterior healing fractures of the left fifth and right fifth, seventh and eighth ribs. Callus is present, suggesting that the fractures are at least 2 weeks old.

Notes

- Non-accidental injury (NAI) needs to be considered in all children who present to the Accident and Emergency department with physical injuries.
- Fifty per cent of cases occur before the age of 1 year.
- Rib fractures are usually multiple, bilateral and posterior.
- The mode of injury is believed to be rib cage compression and distortion during a shaking episode, or during physical blows to the chest.
- Soft callus forms at about 14–21 days.

Hobbs C. Fractures. In: Meadows SR, ed. *ABC of Child Abuse*. 2nd ed. London: BMJ Publishing Group, 1993: 9–13.

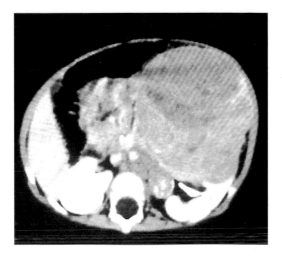

Question

This is a CT of the abdomen.

What are the two most likely diagnoses?

Answers

Neuroblastoma
Wilms' tumour (nephroblastoma)

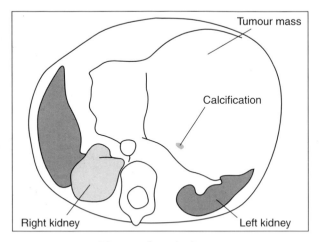

Picture description

The image is taken at the level of the kidneys. There is a large left-sided mass containing areas of calcification. The left kidney is distorted and the para-aortic lymph nodes are enlarged. A neuroblastoma was diagnosed histologically.

Notes

- Neuroblastoma is the commonest extracranial solid tumour, accounting for about 10% of paediatric malignancies.
- Tumours originate from the neural crest and may arise from the sympathetic ganglia and the adrenal medulla.
- Eighty per cent occur in children under 3 years of age.
- About 70% of tumours arise in the abdomen, 20% in the chest.
- Presenting features include a painless abdominal mass, fever, weight loss, anaemia, hepatomegaly and bone pain.
- Fifty per cent of cases will have metastatic disease at presentation.
- Urinary levels of vanilylmandelic acid (VMA) or homovanillic acid (HVA) are raised in 90% of cases.
- Stage IV-S disease is characterized by widespread disease (liver, skin, bone marrow, but not bone cortex) and has a good prognosis.
- Overall survival rate at 10 years is 39%.

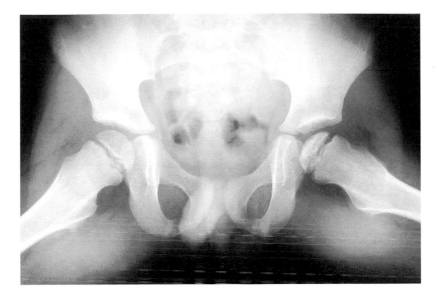

Question

This is a pelvic radiograph of a 5 year old boy.

What is the diagnosis?

Answers

Left-sided Perthes' disease

Perthes' disease
Avascular necrosis of the femoral head

Septic arthritis

Slipped upper femoral epiphyses

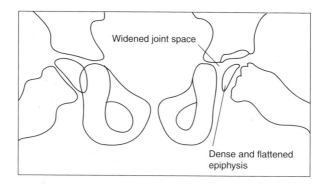

Widened joint space

Dense and flattened epiphysis

Picture description

The left hip joint space is widened. The epiphysis is flattened and dense.

Notes

- Perthes' disease is characterized by idiopathic ischaemic necrosis of the femoral epiphysis.
- Peak age group 3–7 years.
- Male to female ratio 3:1.
- Presenting features: hip or knee pain, limp, limited internal rotation of the hip.
- Bilateral disease occurs in up to 20% of cases.
- The characteristic radiological stages of the disease are:
  (i)   widening of the joint space
  (ii) increase in the bone density of the femoral head with fragmentation and flattening
  (iii) bone reabsorption and new bone formation. The femoral head may be left flattened and widened.
- There is an increased risk of osteoarthritis in adulthood.
- The prognosis is better in girls and younger children.

Wenger DR, Ward WT, Herring JA. Legg–Calvé–Perthes disease. *Journal of Bone and Joint Disease* 1991; **73-A**: 778–88.

Question

This is a cranial ultrasound scan of a 4 day old preterm infant.

What is the diagnosis?

Answers

Grade IV left-sided intraventricular haemorrhage

Intraventricular haemorrhage

Intracranial haemorrhage

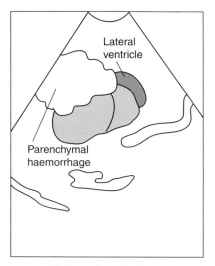

Picture description

The left saggital view is shown. Echogenic blood is seen within the lateral ventricle extending posteriorly into the parenchyma.

Notes

- Intraventricular haemorrhage (IVH) arises from the subependymal germinal matrix, occurring in one-third of infants with a birth weight of less than 1500 g.
- Ninety per cent of cases occur between birth and the fourth day of life.
- Grading:
  - I, subependymal haemorrhage
  - II, intraventricular haemorrhage
  - III, intraventricular haemorrhage with ventricular dilatation
  - IV, parenchymal haemorrhage
- Seventy-five per cent of cases are grade I–II. Most will survive and have no neurological sequelae.
- Grade III/IV haemorrhages are associated with a high mortality rate (50–60%), posthaemorrhagic hydrocephalus and neurodevelopmental impairment.

Questions

This is a skull radiograph of a 3 year old girl.

(a) List two abnormalities.

(b) What single investigation would you perform to confirm your
     diagnosis?

Answers

(a) Copper-beaten skull
Absent sutures

(b) Cranial computed tomogram (CT)

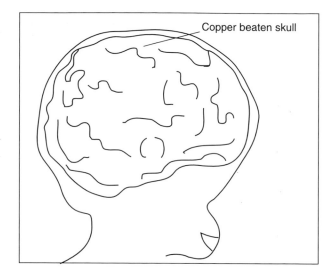

Copper beaten skull

Picture description

The head shape is normal. The lambdoid and coronal sutures are absent. The vault has a copper-beaten appearance. The clinoid processes and sella turcica are normal.

A CT scan of this child's head confirmed the diagnosis of saggital and lambdoid craniosynostosis.

Notes

- The premature closure of a skull suture, craniosynostosis, leads to reduced bone growth in a direction perpendicular to the suture. Various skull deformities result:

  (i) Acrocephaly (tower-like skull) – fusion of the coronal and lambdoid sutures.

  (ii) Scaphocephaly (narrow elongated skull) – fusion of the sagittal suture.

  (iii) Plagiocephaly (asymmetrical skull) – unilateral fusion of the coronal or lambdoid sutures.

- Complications include raised intracranial pressure, breathing difficulties and visual deterioration, especially in children with syndromic craniosynostosis.

- Associated syndromes: Crouzon, Apert and Pfeiffer.
- Surgery for single-suture craniosynostosis is usually definitive and highly successful. It is best performed within the first year of life.
- In complex craniosynostosis, multiple operations will be necessary. Raised intra-cranial pressure must be controlled with vault expansion.

Thompson D, Jones B, Hayward R, Harkness W. Assessment and treatment of craniosynostosis. *British Journal of Hospital Medicine* 1994; **52**: 17–24.

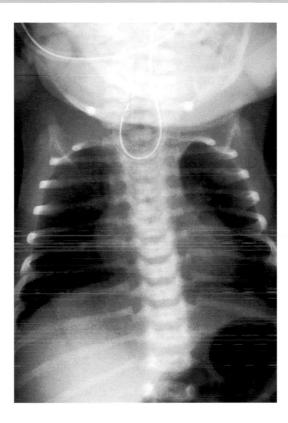

Question

This baby developed respiratory distress at birth.

What is the diagnosis?

Answers

Oesophageal atresia with a distal tracheo-oesophageal fistula
Oesophageal atresia with a tracheo-oesophageal fistula

Oesophageal atresia
Tracheo-oesophageal fistula

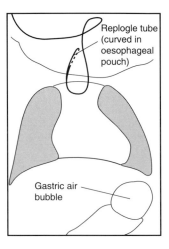

Picture description

A Replogle tube is coiled within the proximal oesophagus. An air-filled stomach establishes the presence of a distal tracheo-oesophageal fistula.

Notes

- The incidence of oesophageal atresia is 1 in 3000. In 80% of cases a distal tracheo-oesophageal fistula is present.
- Clinical features include polyhydramnios, excessive oral secretions, choking, coughing and cyanotic episodes.
- Other malformations are found in 50% of cases, e.g. cardiac defects, duodenal stenosis and imperforate anus. May be part of the VATER/VACTERL syndrome.
- To prevent aspiration infants should be nursed head-up with the oesophageal pouch on continuous suction via a Replogle tube.
- If a primary end-to-end anastomosis is not possible, staged surgical repair is undertaken.
- The long-term survival rate is about 95%, but this decreases to 75% in the presence of other major malformations.
- Long-term problems include gastro-oesophageal reflux, tracheo-malacia, aspiration and strictures.

Examination 4

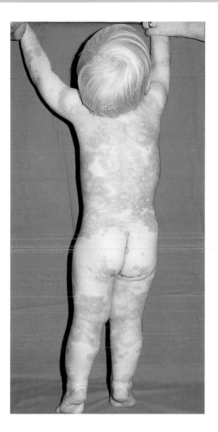

Question

What is the diagnosis?

Answer

Erythema multiforme ✓

Picture description

There are multiple target lesions on the trunk and legs.

Notes

HSV M

- Erythema multiforme is an acute hypersensitivity reaction with characteristic skin lesions and mucosal inflammation.
- Causes include herpes simplex virus, *Mycoplasma pneumoniae*, sulphonamides, penicillins and anticonvulsants.
- There are two subgroups:
  (i)   Symmetrical erythematous macules/papules with superimposed vesicles that evolve into the annular target lesions.
  (ii) Stevens–Johnson syndrome characterized by a severe constitutional disturbance, blistering of mucosal surfaces and target lesions.
- The minor disease is usually self-limiting and is treated symptomatically. Complete healing occurs in 3–4 weeks.
- In severe disease, corticosteroids may be beneficial if started within 2 days of the skin eruption appearing. However, their use is controversial.

Eichenfield LF, Honig PJ. Blistering disorders in childhood. *Pediatric Clinics of North America* 1991; **38**: 959–76.

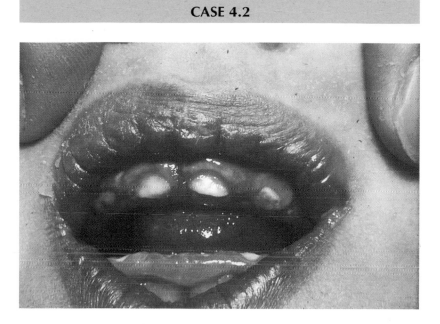

Question

This child had a successful renal transplant two years ago.

What is the most likely cause for the abnormality in this photograph?

Answer

Cyclosporin A therapy

Picture description

Gingival hyperplasia.

Notes

- Hyperplastic gingivitis may occur in patients taking cyclosporin, phenytoin, nifedipine and verapamil.
- Dental plaque is an aetiological factor. Good oral hygiene can prevent the condition.
- Acute leukaemia may be accompanied by generalized enlargement of the gingiva due to infiltration by leukaemic cells.

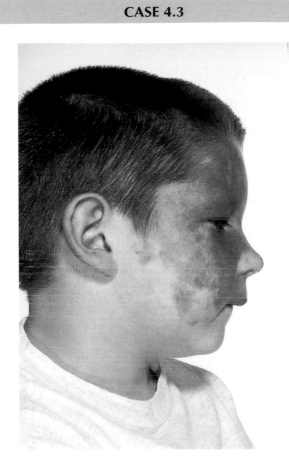

Question

This boy has glaucoma.

What is the diagnosis?

Answer

Sturge–Weber syndrome

Picture description

There is a right-sided port-wine naevus.

Notes

- Sturge–Weber syndrome is defined by a facial port-wine naevus and ipsilateral leptomeningeal haemangiomata.
- Occurs sporadically. Incidence 1 in 50 000 live births.
- Common features include seizures, learning difficulties, buphthalmos and glaucoma.
- The facial naevus is always present at birth and tends to be unilateral, involving the upper face and eyelid, but may also be present on the lower face, trunk and oral mucosa. However, less than 10% of patients with a facial port-wine stain have Sturge–Weber syndrome.
- Occipitoparietal intracranial calcification is found in most patients and characteristically has a curvilinear 'tram line' appearance.
- Seizures develop during the first 3 years of life. They tend to become refractory to anticonvulsants.
- Hemispherectomy can be effective for intractable seizures.
- Regular intraocular pressure monitoring for glaucoma is important.
- Laser therapy is used to minimize the appearance of the port-wine naevus.

Roach ES. Neurocutaneous syndromes. *Pediatric Clinics of North America* 1992; **4**: 591–620.

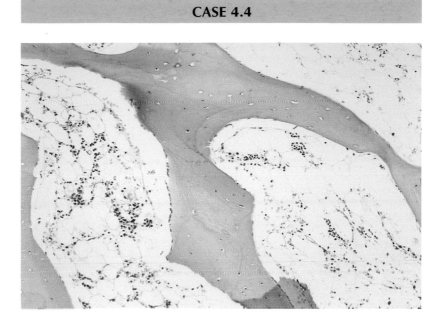

Question

This is a bone marrow trephine from an 11 year old boy who developed pallor and bruising.

What is the most likely diagnosis?

Answers

Acquired aplastic anaemia
Aplastic anaemia

Hypoplastic anaemia

Picture description

The bone marrow is markedly hypocellular with patchy areas of haemopoietic cells. Most of the specimen contains fat cells.

Notes

- Aplastic anaemia, defined as pancytopenia with non-functioning bone marrow, may be acquired or constitutional (Fanconi's).
- Incidence is 1–4 per million children in Europe.
- Acquired aplastic anaemia is usually idiopathic, but can be precipitated by drugs (sulphonamides, non-steroidal anti-inflammatory drugs) and viral infections (hepatitis, Epstein–Barr virus).
- Symptoms include lassitude and weakness due to the anaemia, bleeding as a result of thrombocytopenia, and fever and recurrent infections as a consequence of the neutropenia.
- Patients show a highly variable clinical course. Fifteen per cent die within 3 months of diagnosis, 50% within 15 months.
- Poor prognostic features include a platelet count $<20 \times 10^9/l$, a neutrophil count $<0.2 \times 10^9/l$, a reticulocyte count $<10 \times 10^9/l$, and marked marrow hypocellularity.
- Treatment is supportive with blood transfusions, antibiotics and platelets (only if actively bleeding).
- Bone marrow transplantation with stem cells from histocompatible marrow cures the condition and has a 5 year survival rate of >70%.
- Patients who are not transplanted may benefit from immunosuppression with antithrombocyte globulin or cyclosporin A.

Young NS. Aplastic anaemia. *Lancet* 1995; **346**: 228–32.

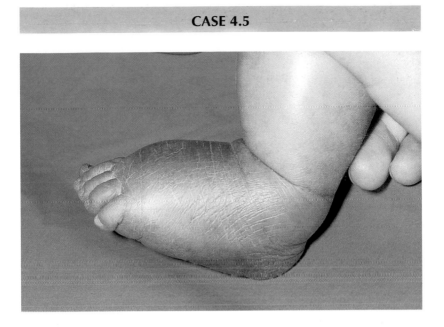

Question

This infant was born at term weighing 1.9 kg.

List the two most likely diagnoses.

Answers

Turner syndrome
45,X karyotype

Noonan syndrome

Congenital nephrotic syndrome

Picture description

There is lymphoedema of the left foot.

Notes

- Turner syndrome has an incidence of 1 in 2500 live female births.
- Approximately 50% of cases have a 45,X karyotype; the rest are a result of mosaicism.
- The clinical phenotype is variable. The common picture is short stature and gonadal dysgenesis.
- Characteristic features at birth include low birth weight and loose skin folds at the nape of the neck. Oedema of the dorsum of the feet is a recognized feature of both Turner and Noonan syndromes.
- Childhood features of Turner syndrome include neck webbing, low hairline, shield-shaped chest with widely spaced nipples, cubitus valgus, pigmented naevi and congenital heart abnormalities (coarctation of the aorta).
- Growth hormone replacement therapy is used to enhance growth.

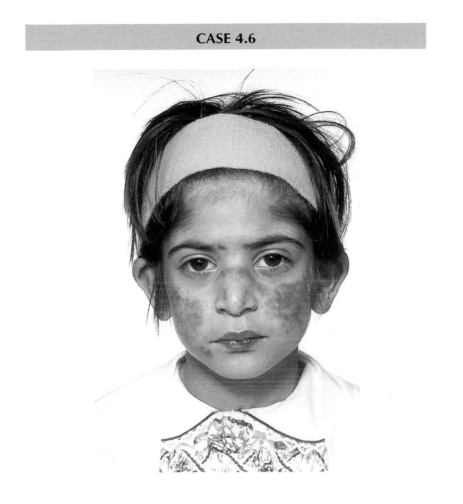

Questions

(a) What is the most likely diagnosis?

(b) What two investigations would you perform to confirm your diagnosis?

Answers

(a)   Systemic lupus erythematosus

Connective tissue disease

(b)   Antinuclear antibodies
Anti-doublestranded DNA antibodies

Autoantibody screen
ESR

Picture description

A classical butterfly rash.

Notes

- Systemic lupus erythematosus (SLE) is an autoimmune multisystem inflammatory disease. It is very uncommon in children.
- Persistent polyclonal B-cell activation results in the widespread tissue deposition of antigen–antibody complexes.
- Presenting features include fever, rash, arthritis and malaise.
- The skin rash can be either a malar butterfly rash or a more generalized polymorphous eruption of the trunk and extremities. The skin lesions may be photosensitive.
- A non-deforming arthritis of the large joint occurs in 25% of cases.
- Progressive renal failure is the leading cause of death. Focal segmental glomerulonephritis usually responds to steroids.
- Central nervous system disease is varied and may include fits, behavioural changes, coma, hemiplegia and focal neuropathies.
- Antinuclear antibodies are usually present, but not diagnostic. Anti-dsDNA antibodies are very specific for SLE but not always present in mild disease.
- C3 complement levels are low in active disease, especially with nephritis.
- Treatment options include high-dose oral corticosteroids, azathioprine and cyclophosphamide.
- With early treatment, the 5 year survival rate is 95%.

Cervera R *et al.* Systemic lupus erythematosus: clinical and immunological patterns of disease expression in a cohort of 1000 patients. The European Working Party on Systemic Lupus Erythematosus. *Medicine* 1993; **72**: 113–24.

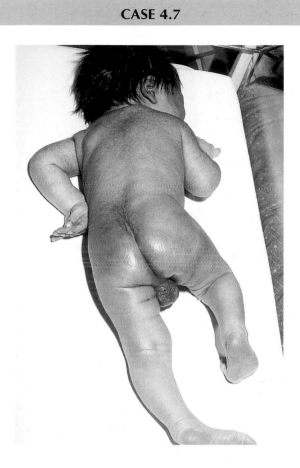

Question

What is the diagnosis?

Answer

Mongolian blue spot

Picture description

There is a large blue-black macule overlying the lumbosacral region, buttocks and upper thighs.

Notes

- A mongolian blue spot is a dermal melanocytic naevus.
- Commonest in Asian and Afro-Caribbean infants.
- Usually fades during infancy, but some lesions do persist into adulthood.
- No treatment is required.

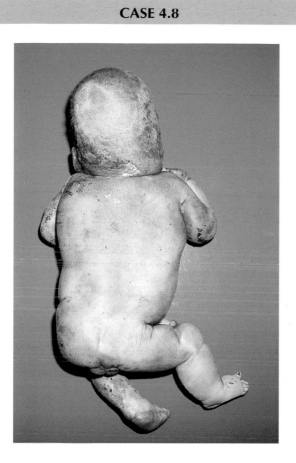

Question

What is this condition?

Answer

Hydrops fetalis

Picture description

Oedematous stillborn infant.

Notes

- Hydrops fetalis is categorized into two groups:
  - (i) **Immunological** – secondary to anaemia following maternal isoimmunization against rhesus or other red cell antigens.
  - (ii) **Non-immunological** – the majority of cases. Commonest causes are chromosomal abnormalities, cardiac defects, pulmonary abnormalities, infection and multiple births.
- Up to 85% of cases are of unknown aetiology.
- The hydropic fetus or newborn infant will have widespread subcutaneous oedema, pleural effusions, ascites and an oedematous placenta.
- The diagnosis can be made on antenatal ultrasonography.
- Pulmonary hypoplasia is present in 90% of cases.
- At delivery, most babies require intubation and ventilation with high pressure. Thoracentesis, abdominal paracentesis and pericardiocentesis may be indicated.

Stephenson T, Zucollo J, Mohajer M. Diagnosis and management of non-immune hydrops in the newborn. *Archives of Disease in Childhood* 1994; **70**: F151–4.

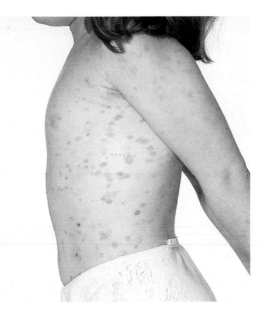

Question

What is this skin condition?

Answers

Guttate psoriasis
Discoid psoriasis

Psoriasis

Picture description

There are multiple pink, scaly macules distributed predominantly on the trunk.

Notes

- Psoriasis is not uncommon in children. About 25% of patients develop the condition before their 16th birthday.
- Guttate psoriasis:
  - usually occurs in adolescents.
  - often follows a beta-haemolytic streptococcal or viral infection.
  - most children do not develop chronic psoriasis.
  - topical corticosteroids are the mainstay of treatment.
  - ultraviolet light and tar preparations are alternative therapies.

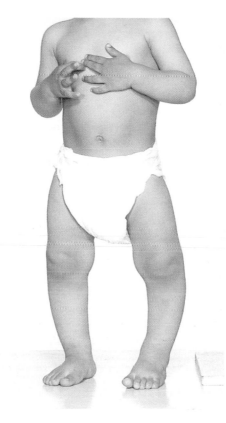

Questions

(a) What is the diagnosis?

(b) List the two most likely causes of this condition.

Answers

(a) Rickets

Bowed legs
Genu varum

(b) Lack of exposure to sunlight
Prolonged breast feeding and maternal vitamin D deficiency
Nutritional deficiency of vitamin D

Picture description

This Asian child has bowed legs.

Notes

- Classical rickets is due to vitamin D deficiency. The mineralization of bone is defective.
- Clinical features: craniotabes, genus varum, rib cage rosary.
- The common radiographic findings are cupping, splaying and fraying of the metaphysis.
- The commonest causes of vitamin D deficiency in Asian children is lack of exposure to sunlight and poor dietary intake.
- Oral vitamin D administration will produce healing on radiography after 2–4 weeks.
- Secondary causes include:
  - (i)   Renal disease (defective 1-hydroxylation).
  - (ii)   Liver disease (defective 25-hydroxylation).
  - (iii) Malabsorption of vitamin D.
  - (iv)   Hepatic enzyme induction, e.g. by anticonvulsants.
  - (v)   Familial hypophosphataemic rickets (vitamin D resistance).
  - (vi)   Tubular dysfunction, e.g. renal tubular acidosis, Fanconi's syndrome.

Question

List two possible diagnoses.

Answers

Right-sided periorbital cellulitis

Right-sided orbital cellulitis

Picture description

The right eyelid and periorbital tissues are swollen and inflamed.

Notes

Orbital cellulitis
- An inflammation of the orbit with proptosis, limitation of eye movements and oedema of the conjunctiva (chemosis).
- Infection may result directly from a wound or via haematological spread.
- The most common organisms are *Staphylococcus aureus*, group A beta-haemolytic streptococci, *Streptococcus pneumoniae* and *Haemophilus influenzae* (prior to the introduction of the Hib vaccination programme).
- Prompt and aggressive treatment with intravenous antibiotics is important. Potential complications include cavernous sinus thrombosis, meningitis and brain abscess.

Periorbital cellulitis
- An inflammation of the eyelid and surrounding tissues *without* proptosis, limitation of eye movements or chemosis.
- This condition is common in young children and may result from trauma or an infected wound.
- Without appropriate antibiotic therapy it may progress to a true orbital cellulitis.

Weiss A, Friendly D, Eglin K, Chang M, Gold B. Bacterial periorbital and orbital cellulitis in childhood. *Ophthalmology* 1983; **90**: 195–203.

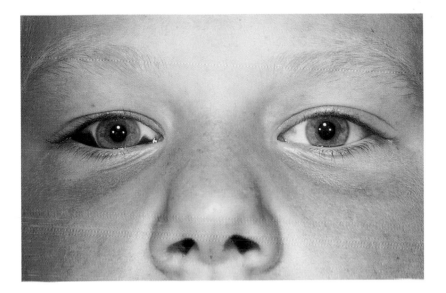

Question

Give two possible diagnoses.

Answers

Whooping cough
Non-accidental injury

Clotting disorder
Bleeding disorder
Trauma

Picture description

There are right-sided subconjunctival haemorrhages.

Notes

- Whooping cough is caused by the Gram-negative bacilli *Bordetella pertussis* and *Bordetella parapertussis*.
- Transmission is by droplet spread.
- The incubation period is usually 7–14 days.
- There are three identifiable phases to the disease:
  - (i) The *catarrhal* phase with coryza and a dry cough.
  - (ii) The *paroxysmal* phase with bouts of coughing and the characteristic inspiratory whoop at the end of each paroxysm. The whoop is not found in infants.
  - (iii) The *convalescent* phase with gradual improvement in symptoms. The cough can persist for several months.
- Very young children may present with apnoea alone.
- There is no cross-immunity between the different organisms.
- Complications include conjunctival haemorrhages, convulsions, epistaxis, pneumonia and bronchiectasis.
- Erythromycin is used to prevent further transmission and usually renders a sufferer non-infectious within 5 days.

Question

The mother of this newborn infant was concerned about the appearance of her baby's palate.

What is the diagnosis?

Answers

Epstein's pearls
Gingival cysts of the newborn

Picture description

There are multiple white cysts in the midline of the palate.

Notes

- Epstein's pearls are keratin-containing cysts occurring on the palate or alveolar mucosa in 80% of newborns.
- They cause no symptoms and disappear spontaneously after a few weeks.

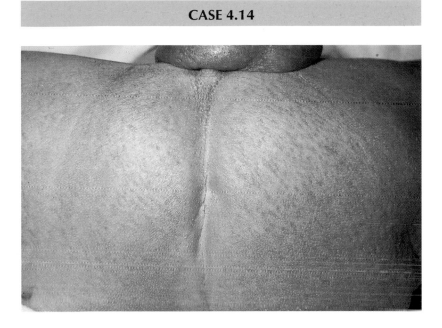

Question

What is the diagnosis?

Answer

Imperforate anus

Notes

- Anorectal malformations have an incidence of 1 in 5000 live births.
- Associated anomalies (genitourinary, cardiac, vertebral, alimentary) are found in 50% of cases.
- Malformations can be classified according to their relationship to the puborectalis component of the levator ani muscles. High lesions lie above the levator sling, intermediate on the sling, and low lesions below the sling.
- A fistula is present with imperforate anus in 90% of cases. The commonest types are rectourethral in males and rectovestibular in females.
- An obvious abnormality may be discovered during the newborn examination. Alternatively, the infant may present with intestinal obstruction, meconium in the urine or with a meconium-discharging fistula.
- Low malformations are more common in girls. Generally, they do not require a colostomy and definitive surgery can be undertaken during the first few days of life.
- High and intermediate malformations are more common in boys. A colostomy is required prior to surgical reconstruction during the first year of life.
- Complications of surgery include anal strictures, recurrent fistulae and urinary incontinence.
- The outlook for faecal continence is excellent in low malformations. High malformations are more problematic, especially in the presence of sacral abnormalities.

Peña A. Imperforate anus and cloacal malformations. In: Ashcraft KW, Holder TM, eds. *Pediatric Surgery*. 2nd ed. Philadelphia: WB Saunders, 1993: 372–92.

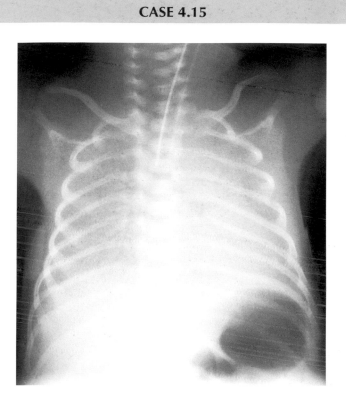

Question

What is the diagnosis?

Answers

Hyaline membrane disease
Respiratory distress syndrome
Group B haemolytic streptococcal infection
Congenital pneumonia
Aspiration pneumonia

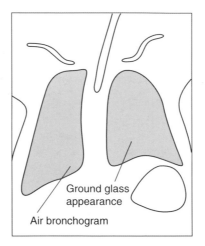

Picture description

The infant is intubated. There is a diffuse, fine granular (ground glass) appearance to the lung fields, with an air bronchogram in the lower right zone. The cardiac borders are obscured.

Notes

- Surfactant is produced from 22 to 24 weeks' gestation onwards by type II pneumocytes. There is a surge in production at 35 weeks.
- Up to 70% of infants of under 32 weeks' gestation will suffer from hyaline membrane disease (HMD).
- Predisposing factors for HMD: prematurity, maternal diabetes, male sex, elective caesarean section, perinatal asphyxia and hypothermia.
- Protecting factors against HMD: intrauterine growth retardation, maternal drug abuse, prolonged rupture of membranes and antenatal corticosteroids.
- Group B haemolytic streptococcal infection can have an identical clinical picture to HMD.
- Surfactant therapy improves oxygenation and reduces the incidence of pneumothorax.

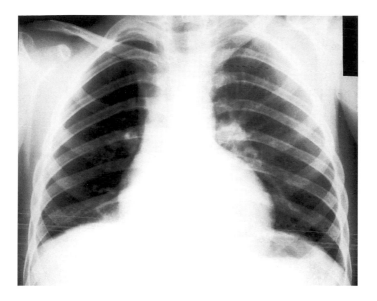

Question

List three abnormalities on this chest radiograph.

Answers

Right lower lobe collapse
Mediastinal deviation to the right
Small right lung field
Hyperlucent right lung field
Depressed right hilum

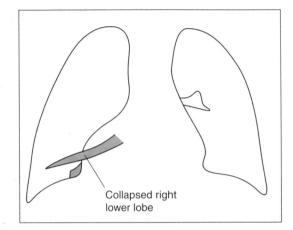

Collapsed right
lower lobe

Picture description

The abnormalities are the result of a right lower lobe collapse. The collapsed lobe is seen as a 'triangle' opacity behind the heart shadow. There is compensatory overinflation of the right upper and middle lobes. The outline of the medial aspect of the hemidiaphragm is blurred.

Notes

- Lobar collapse is not uncommon in infants and children, and results from external compression of the airways, intraluminal obstruction (e.g. foreign body), or reduced respiratory effort (e.g. during anaesthesia).
- The right middle lobe is prone to external compression from the lymph nodes that surround its bronchus. In right middle lobe collapse, the right heart border is obscured.

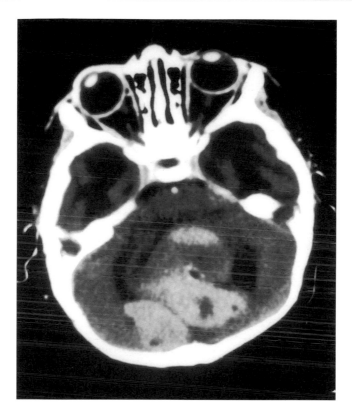

Question

This 1 year old boy presented with vomiting. A cranial CT was performed.

What is the diagnosis?

Answers

Primary cerebellar tumour
Medulloblastoma
Astrocytoma

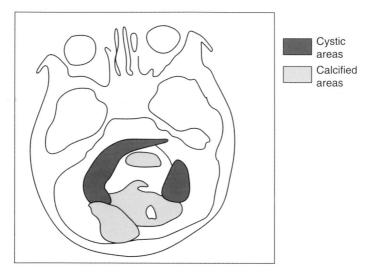

Legend:
- ■ Cystic areas
- ☐ Calcified areas

Picture description

There is a large cystic, calcified mass within the posterior fossa with gross hydrocephalus. A diagnosis of medulloblastoma was made histologically.

Notes

- Primary central nervous system tumours are the commonest solid tumours in childhood. Peak age 5–9 years.
- Approximately 50% are found infratentorially in children over 1 year of age.
- There are two main histological types: glial cell tumours (astrocytoma, ependymoma) and primitive neuroectodermal tumours (medulloblastoma).
- Symptoms and signs of raised intracranial pressure (headache, nausea, vomiting, diplopia, papilloedema) are generally found with posterior fossa tumours, whereas focal neurological signs are associated with supratentorial tumours.
- The initial management is surgery to establish a histological diagnosis and to reduce the tumour bulk. Subsequent treatment is with radiotherapy and chemotherapy.

- Cerebellar astrocytomas comprise about 30–40% of posterior fossa tumours. Most are composed of cystic and solid tissue and are histologically benign. The prognosis is good, with a 5 year survival rate of 90%.
- The medulloblastoma is the second most common posterior fossa tumour, representing 20–30% of all childhood brain tumours. Five year survival rate is 42%.
- Long-term sequelae of treatment for brain tumours include cognitive impairment and endocrine deficiencies. Second malignancies occur in about 1% of patients.

Pollack IF. Brain tumours in children. *New England Journal of Medicine* 1994; **331**: 1500–7.

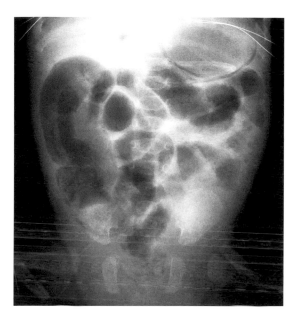

Questions

This premature infant underwent open heart surgery for complex congenital heart disease.

(a) List three radiological abnormalities on this abdominal radiograph.

(b) What is the diagnosis?

Answers

(a) Pneumotosis intestinalis/intramural gas
Gaseous bowel distension
Gas within the portal system
Thickened bowel wall

(b) Neonatal necrotizing enterocolitis

Bowel obstruction

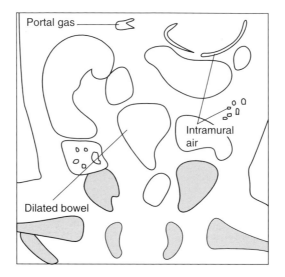

Picture description

Air is seen in the wall of the stomach as linear translucent streaks. Intramural bubbles of gas give the bowel a 'frothy' appearance.

Notes

- Necrotizing enterocolitis is primarily a disease of the very low birth weight infant (<1.5 kg), although about 10% of cases occur in term infants.
- Incidence 0.5 to 15 per 1000 live births.
- Multiple aetiological factors include infection, hypoxia, hypovolaemia, umbilical catheterization and exchange transfusion. Breast milk is protective.
- Clinical features: lethargy, hypotonia, apnoea, abdominal distension, bloody stools and vomiting (with or without bile).
- Medical treatment: cessation of feeds, correction of hypovolaemia, anaemia, coagulopathy and acidosis, broad-spectrum antibiotics,

nasogastric drainage, total parenteral nutrition and mechanical ventilation if required.

- Deterioration despite maximal medical treatment and bowel perforation are indications for surgical intervention.
- Mortality rate is between 20 and 40%. Poor prognostic factors include birth weight <1.5 kg, disseminated intravascular coagulation and bacteraemia.
- Complications include recurrence (10% within 1 month of the initial presentation), strictures, malabsorption and the short gut syndrome.

Lucas A, Cole TJ. Breast milk and neonatal necrotising enterocolitis. *Lancet* 1990; **336**: 1519–23.

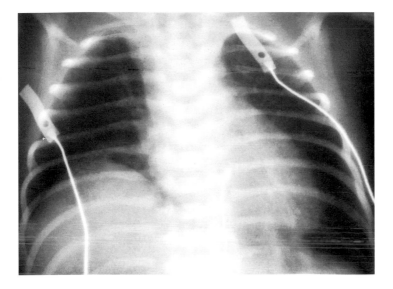

Question

This infant of 35 weeks gestation was ventilated at birth for hyaline membrane disease. Following extubation at 72 hours of age he developed increasing respiratory distress.

What is the most likely cause for this deterioration?

Answers

Right diaphragmatic eventration

Diaphragmatic eventration
Raised right hemidiaphragm

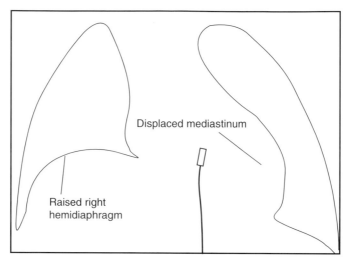

Displaced mediastinum

Raised right
hemidiaphragm

Picture description

ECG leads and an umbilical arterial catheter are *in situ*. The mediastinum is slightly displaced to the left. The right hemidiaphragm is elevated.

Notes

- Diaphragmatic eventration may be congenital (non-paralytic) or acquired (paralytic), secondary to damage to the phrenic nerve at birth.
- An Erb's or Klumpke's palsy usually coexists when the defect is acquired during delivery.
- In the congenital form:
  - (i)   There is a defect in the development of the central tendon of the diaphragm.
  - (ii)   The defect may be focal or affect the entire diaphragm.
  - (iii) The condition is usually unilateral, more commonly affecting the left side.
- A focal eventration may be asymptomatic.
- A large defect will present with respiratory distress at birth. The mediastinum will be shifted to the contralateral side and the abdomen may be scaphoid. The differential diagnosis includes diaphragmatic

hernia, congenital lung cyst and cystic adenomatoid malformation.

- Paradoxical movements of the diaphragm during inspiration and expiration may be seen on fluoroscopic or ultrasonographic examination.
- Asymptomatic infants do not require treatment. In the symptomatic infant, diaphragmatic plication does not always improve function. Pulmonary hypoplasia may limit any clinical benefit.

Question

This is a micturating cystourethrogram performed on a 3 month old boy.

What is the diagnosis?

Answers

Congenital posterior urethral valves
Posterior urethral valves

Vesicoureteric reflux

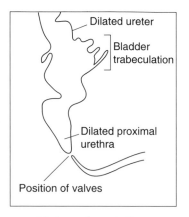

Picture description

The proximal urethra is dilated with a convex lower border representing the position of posterior urethral valves. There is bladder trabeculation and dilatation of the right ureter.

Notes

- Posterior urethral valves occur only in boys and is the commonest cause of acute urinary obstruction during the first year of life.
- Hydronephrosis, vesicoureteric reflux and renal impairment develop antenatally.
- If not detected on antenatal ultrasonography, the child presents within the first few months of life with failure to thrive, poor urinary stream or renal failure.
- Hyponatraemia and metabolic acidosis are common.
- Initial management involves bladder drainage with an indwelling catheter, intravenous fluids, oral sodium bicarbonate solution and antibiotics.
- Valves are resected using endoscopic transurethral techniques. In a small infant, a cutaneous vesicostomy allows valve resection to be delayed.
- Impaired renal function is common, with 7% progressing to end-stage renal failure.

Gough DCS. The dilated urinary system. In: Postlethwaite RJ, ed. *Clinical Paediatric Nephrology*. 2nd ed. Oxford: Butterworth–Heinemann, 1994: 345–57.

Examination 5

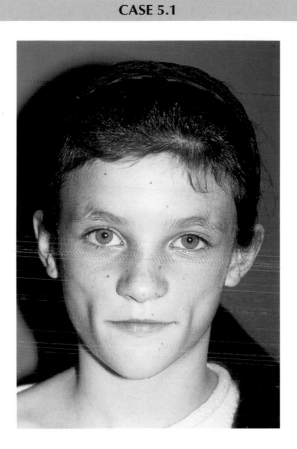

Question

This 12 year old girl was found to have a random blood glucose level of 9 mmol/l.

What is the most likely diagnosis?

Answers

Partial lipodystrophy

Lipodystrophy

Picture description

This girl has a very thin, wasted appearance as a result of the loss of facial subcutaneous fat.

Notes

- Classical partial lipodystrophy involves the symmetrical loss of subcutaneous fat from the face. The arms and upper trunk may be affected, but the lower trunk and legs are spared.
- The male to female ratio is 1:4.
- The cause is unknown.
- Onset is usually during the first decade of life.
- Abnormal glucose intolerance is common and is thought to be secondary to insulin resistance. Approximately 20% of cases develop clinical diabetes.
- C3 and C3 nephritic factor levels are low.
- Patients may develop type II mesangiocapillary glomerulonephritis.

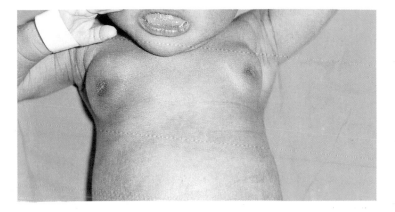

Question

What is the diagnosis?

Answers

Neonatal mastitis
Mastitis neonatorum

Bilateral breast enlargement

Picture description

Bilateral breast enlargement with a white discharge from the right nipple.

Notes

- During the neonatal period breast enlargement is common in babies of both sexes.
- Transplacental passage of maternal hormones leads to breast tissue hyperplasia with milk secretion.
- Attempts to empty the breast by massage will increase milk production.
- The condition resolves after the first week of life.

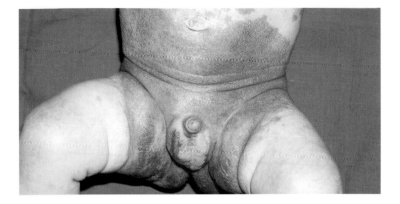

Question

What is the diagnosis?

Answers

Candidiasis

Nappy rash
Psoriasis

Picture description

There is a diffuse erythematous rash in the nappy area with peripheral satellite lesions.

Notes

- Candidiasis is a common cause of nappy rash. Oral thrush is often present at the same time.
- Management: topical antifungal agents (nystatin and miconazole), frequent nappy changes and the treatment of oral disease.

Questions

This blood film is from a 5 year old boy who presented with pallor.

(a) List three abnormalities.

(b) What is the most likely diagnosis?

Answers

(a) Microcytosis
Hypochromia
Anisocytosis
Poikilocytosis

(b) Iron deficiency anaemia
Microcytic anaemia

Picture description

The mean cell volume on this film is 51 fl. There are variations in the cell diameter (anisocytosis) and cell shape (poikilocytosis). Elongated erythrocytes (pencil poikilocytes) are present.

Notes

- Iron deficiency anaemia is the commonest childhood nutritional deficiency and results from inadequate intake, increased requirements with accelerating growth, reduced intestinal absorption, and blood loss.
- The diagnosis is made from a microcytic, hypochromic blood film with decreased ferritin and increased free erythrocyte protoporphyrin.
- Preventive measures include:
  (i) Avoiding cow's milk during the first year of life as it is a poor source of iron. Breast feeding or an iron-fortified formula is recommended during this time.
  (ii) Weaning, at 4 months and not later than 6 months, with iron-rich or iron-fortified foods.
  (iii) Introduction of vitamin C containing foods into the diet to increase iron absorption.
  (iv) Iron supplementation for low birth weight and premature infants.
- Failure to respond to oral iron supplements may suggest poor compliance, malabsorption, persistent blood loss or an incorrect diagnosis.

Auckett A. *Iron Deficiency in Children. Clinical Opinion.* London: BPA, March 1996.

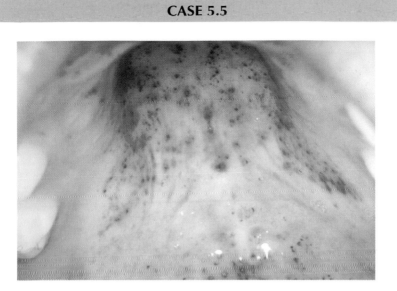

Question

This 10 year old girl presented with a history of fever and cervical lymphadenopathy.

What is the most likely diagnosis?

Answers

Infectious mononucleosis
Glandular fever
Epstein–Barr virus infection

Acute leukaemia

Picture description

Submucosal haemorrhages on the palate.

Notes

- Infectious mononucleosis is caused by the Epstein–Barr virus (EBV).
- Spread is by droplet infection.
- The incubation period is 4–6 weeks.
- The characteristic clinical triad is sore throat, lymphadenopathy and splenomegaly.
- In infants and young children the condition is often mild.
- Laboratory findings: atypical lymphocytes, positive Paul–Bunnell heterophile antibody test (60%), raised EBV-specific IgM titres, abnormal liver function tests.
- Complications include hepatitis, aseptic meningitis, Guillain–Barré syndrome, encephalitis, autoimmune haemolytic anaemia, thrombocytopenia, upper airway obstruction and splenic rupture.
- Management is mainly supportive. A short course of steroids may give symptomatic relief from airway obstruction secondary to lymphadenopathy.

Question

What is the most likely mode of injury?

Answers

Non-accidental scald
Non-accidental injury
Forced immersion in hot water

Scalding

Picture description

There is a large scald on the right foot. It has a stocking distribution with a clear tidemark. The remaining skin is white and soggy.

Notes

- Scalds are caused by hot water, food and drinks. They may be accidental or non-accidental.
- The depth of the burn depends on the temperature and duration of exposure to the heat source.
- Scalded skin is blistered, peeling, soggy and blanched.
- In physical abuse, scalds may have a glove and stocking distribution without splash marks. There may be a delay in seeking medical advice.
- To punish soiling or wetting, a child's buttocks may be immersed into a bath of hot water. The 'hole in doughnut' burn is characteristic, with sparing of the skin that is pressed on to the base of the bath.

Hobbs, C. Burns and scalds. In: Meadows SR, ed. *ABC of Child Abuse.* 2nd ed. London: BMJ Publishing Group, 1993: 20–3.

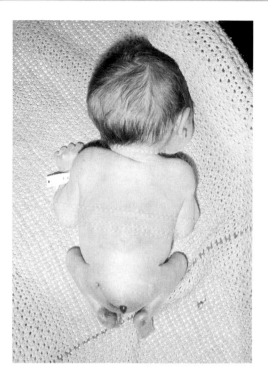

Question

What is the underlying abnormality?

Answers

Lumbosacral agenesis

Sacral agenesis

Picture description

This baby's lumbar sacral region is abnormal. The buttocks are narrow and dimpled, with a horizontal patulous anus. The hips and knees are flexed with bilateral talipes equinovarus.

Notes

- Lumbosacral agenesis is commoner in infants of diabetic mothers.
- The type of deformity ranges from partial sacral or coccygeal agenesis to complete lumbosacral agenesis.
- Clinical features include hypotonic paraplegia and an atonic bladder.
- Scoliosis, hemivertebrae and spina bifida are associated anomalies.
- Patients with an intact sacropelvic ring are able to learn to walk.

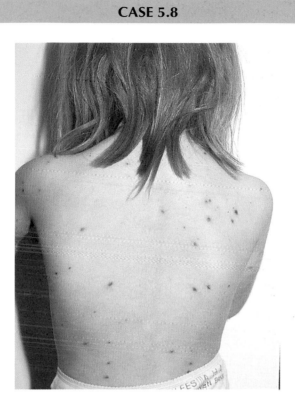

Question

What is the diagnosis?

Answer

Chickenpox

Picture description

Multiple, small encrusted vesicles.

Notes

- The varicella zoster virus is transmitted by direct contact or droplet infection.
- The incubation period is 10–21 days.
- A short coryzal illness is followed by fever and an itchy vesicular rash.
- The rash initially appears over the trunk and then spreads to the limbs.
- Complications include staphylococcal skin infections, hepatitis, thrombocytopenia, arthritis, cerebellar ataxia, post-infective polyneuropathy and encephalitis.
- Period of infectivity: 1–2 days prior to the rash appearing until the lesions are encrusted.
- Varicella zoster immunoglobulin (ZIG) should be given to the newborn if the mother has developed chickenpox in the 7 days before or after birth.

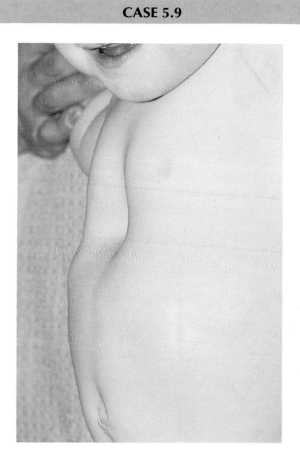

Question

What is the diagnosis?

Answers

Pectus excavatum
Funnel chest

Chest deformity

Notes

- Pectus excavatum is the commonest congenital chest deformity and results from abnormal costal cartilages.
- It occurs sporadically and is associated with Marfan's syndrome.
- Male to female ratio is 3:1.
- Clinical features include decreased anteroposterior diameter of the chest, thoracolumbar kyphosis and rounded shoulders.
- Most patients are asymptomatic; impaired cardiopulmonary function is rare.
- Chest wall remodelling is performed in symptomatic patients and in those with severe deformities.
- Silicone implants may be used for milder abnormalities.

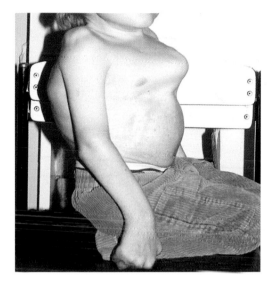

Question

What is the diagnosis?

Answers

Morquio's syndrome
Morquio–Brailsford syndrome
Mucopolysaccharidosis type IV

Mucopolysaccharidosis

Severe kyphoscoliosis
Congenital chest deformity

Picture description

This boy has a short neck and trunk, kyphoscoliosis and severe pectus carinatum.

Notes

- Morquio's syndrome, type IV mucopolysaccharidosis, is due to the defective catabolism of keratan sulphate and chondroitin sulphate.
- Two forms of the disease have been described:
  (i)   Type A (classical) – deficiency of N-acetylgalactosamine 6-sulphate sulphatase.
  (ii) Type B (mild form) – deficiency of β-galactosidase.
- The main features are severe skeletal deformity, dwarfism with thoracolumbar gibbus and pectus carinatum.
- Joint laxity and short stature appear at about 1 year of age.
- Corneal clouding and deafness develop later in life.
- Intellect is normal or slightly impaired.
- Keratan sulphate is excreted in the urine.
- Death usually occurs in the third or fourth decade of life from cor pulmonale.

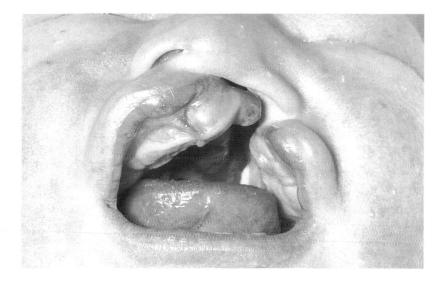

Question

What is the diagnosis?

Answers

Left-sided cleft lip and palate

Cleft lip and palate
Cleft lip

Notes

- Cleft lip and/or palate (CL/P) has an incidence of 1 in 600 live births in the UK.
- Ultrasonographic diagnosis of cleft lip *in utero* is possible from about 17 weeks' gestation.
- Associations: trisomies 13 and 18, Pierre Robin sequence, Di George sequence, EEC (ectrodactyly, ectodermal dysplasia, CL/P), Goldenhar and fetal phenytoin syndromes.
- Recurrence risk of cleft palate alone is 2%, whereas CL/P has a 4% risk. In familial cases, the risk for subsequent offspring is 10% when a sibling and parent are affected.
- Problems include impaired facial growth, dental abnormalities, feeding difficulties, speech disorders, hearing impairment and psychological difficulties.
- Lip repair is undertaken at 3 months and palate repair between 6 and 12 months of age.

Habel A, Sell D, Mars M. Management of cleft lip and palate. *Archives of Disease in Childhood* 1996; **74**: 360–6.

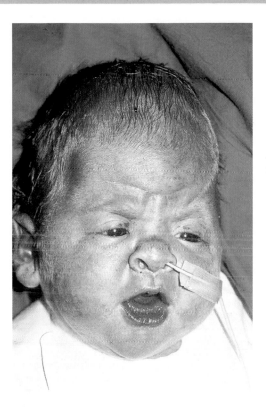

Questions

(a) List the two most likely diagnoses.

(b) How can you distinguish between them?

Answers

(a) Apert syndrome
Crouzon syndrome

Acrocephaly
Craniosynostosis

(b) Children with Apert syndrome have syndactyly

Picture description

This child with Apert syndrome has a very prominent forehead, midfacial hypoplasia hypertelorism and a nasogastric tube *in situ.* His hands and feet display syndactyly.

Notes

- Apert syndrome is characterized by craniosynostosis, midfacial hypoplasia and symmetrical syndactyly.
- Inheritance is autosomal dominant, with most cases representing new mutations.
- Incidence 1 in 160 000 live births.
- Acrocephaly results from fusion of the coronal, saggital and, less commonly, the lambdoid sutures.
- Syndactyly commonly involves the second, third and fourth fingers.
- The majority of patients have learning difficulties.
- Otitis media is common and is related to the high frequency of cleft palate.
- The orbits are shallow leading to proptosis. Patients are at risk of eye trauma.

Cohen MM, Kreiborg S. An updated paediatric perspective on the Apert syndrome. *American Journal of Diseases of Children* 1993; **147**: 989–93.

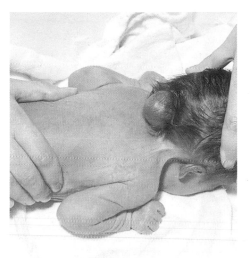

Question

What is the diagnosis?

Answers

Occipital encephalocele/meningocele

Lipoma
Tumour

Picture description

There is a smooth saccular swelling protruding from the occipital region.

Notes

- Encephaloceles are herniations of brain and meninges through a midline defect in the skull.
- Incidence ranges from 1:5000 to 1:9000 live births.
- The majority of encephaloceles occur in the occipital area (75%).
- Encephaloceles may be identified on fetal ultrasonography.
- Alpha-fetoprotein levels are raised in amniotic fluid if there is an open defect.
- There is an increased risk of hydrocephalus due to aqueduct stenosis or a Chiari malformation.
- Patients are at risk of visual impairment, focal motor weakness, spasticity and seizures.
- The recurrence risk in siblings is approximately 3%.

Brown MS, Sheridan-Pereira M. Outlook for the child with a cephalocele. *Pediatrics* 1992; **90**: 914–19.

Question

What is the most likely diagnosis?

Answer

Non-accidental injury

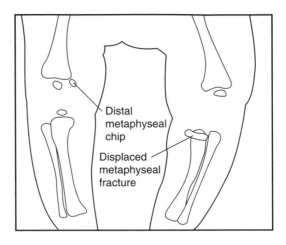

Picture description

There is a metaphyseal fracture of the left proximal tibia and a chip fracture on the medial aspect of the right distal femoral metaphysis.

Notes

- Radiographic features suggestive of NAI include:
  - multiple fractures of different ages
  - metaphyseal–epiphyseal injuries
  - rib fractures
  - subperiosteal new bone formation
- Metaphyseal and epiphyseal fractures result from acceleration and declaration as the infant is shaken by the body, arms or legs.
- Rib fractures are often multiple, bilateral and posterior, and are believed to result from compression and shaking of the thoracic cage.

Hobbs C. Fractures. In: Meadows SR, ed. *ABC of Child Abuse.* 2nd ed. London: BMJ Publishing Group, 1993: 9–13.

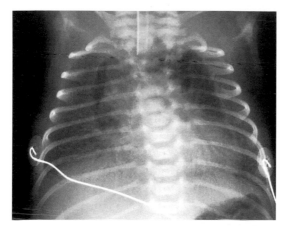

Question

This newborn preterm infant was ventilated shortly after birth because of hyaline membrane disease.

What is the additional diagnosis?

Answers

Pneumomediastinum

Pneumothorax
Lung cyst

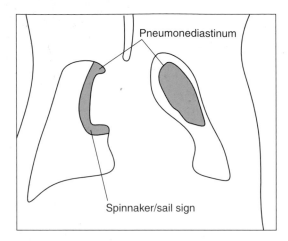

Pneumonediastinum

Spinnaker/sail sign

Picture description

An endotracheal tube and heart monitor leads are *in situ*. Air is present within the superior mediastinum, lifting the thymus away from the pericardium to give the 'spinnaker' or 'sail' sign. A pneumothorax is excluded by the presence of lung markings in the peripheral lung fields.

Notes

- Pneumomediastinum has an incidence of 2.5 per 1000 live births.
- Over 90% of cases are asymptomatic. Severe respiratory distress is rare.
- They are more common in term than in preterm infants.
- Risk factors include postmaturity, meconium aspiration syndrome and air leaks, such as pneumothoraces and pulmonary interstitial emphysema.
- Drainage is not possible as the air is loculated.

Question

This 14 month old girl was tender above her right eye.

What is the most likely diagnosis?

Answer

Langerhans' cell histiocytosis

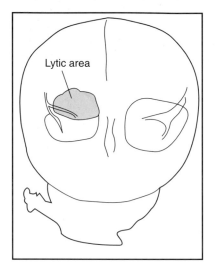

Picture description

There is a sharply demarcated lytic defect overlying the right superior orbital margin which is characteristic of Langerhans' cell histiocytosis.

Notes

- Langerhans' cell histiocytosis is a reactive proliferative disease characterized by the accumulation of abnormal histiocytes.
- Incidence 2–5 per million, peaking between 1 and 4 years.
- Clinical presentation ranges from isolated lesions in skin or bone to multiorgan involvement.
- Bone lesions are found in almost all patients presenting with tenderness, pain and swelling. The skull, femur and ribs are the most frequently affected sites.
- Patients with localized disease (skin or bone) have a good prognosis. Treatment may be unnecessary as in many cases the lesions regress spontaneously.
- Multiorgan involvement, particularly in children under 2 years old, carries a poor prognosis. Cytotoxic/steroid therapy appears to benefit patients with multiorgan involvement.

Egeler RM, D'Angio GJ. Langerhans cell histiocytosis. *Journal of Pediatrics* 1995; **127**: 1-11.

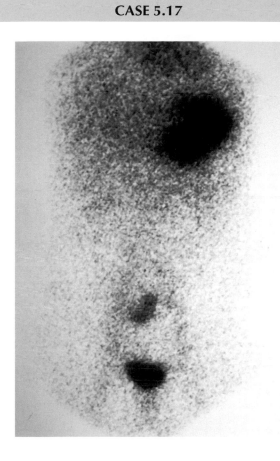

Questions

This 3 year old child presented with rectal bleeding.

(a) What is the investigation?

(b) What is the most likely diagnosis?

Answers

(a) ^{99m}Technetium radioisotope scan

     Isotope scan

     Meckel's scan

(b)   Meckel's diverticulum

     Duplicated bowel segment

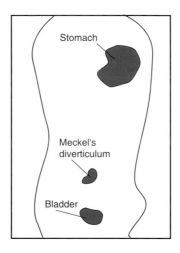

Picture description

As technetium has an affinity for parietal cells the scan is used to identify ectopic gastric mucosa. The isotope is excreted via the kidneys. The stomach and bladder are visualized, with a third 'hot spot' above the bladder representing a Meckel's diverticulum.

Notes

- A Meckel's diverticulum is a remnant of the vitellointestinal duct, arising from the free border of the ileum 40–100 cm proximal to the ileocaecal valve.
- It is found in about 2% of the population, but symptomatic in only 1 in 3000.
- Up to half contain acid-secreting gastric mucosa.
- A diverticulum may become inflamed, haemorrhage, perforate or cause an intussusception.
- Bleeding is more common in preschool children.
- Diverticolectomy is performed in symptomatic cases.

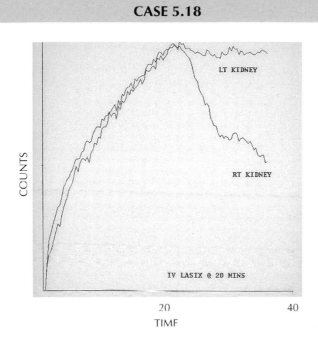

COUNTS

LT KIDNEY

RT KIDNEY

IV LASIX @ 20 MINS

20   40

TIME

Questions

This child presented with a history of left loin pain. A ⁹⁹ᵐTc-labelled diethylene triamine penta-acetic acid (DTPA) scan was performed.

(a) Describe the scan finding.

(b) What is the underlying diagnosis?

Answers

(a)   Prolonged transit time of left kidney with no response to frusemide

Isotope retention by the left kidney

(b)   Left-sided pelviureteric junction obstruction

Pelviureteric junction obstruction

Obstructive uropathy

Picture description

This isotope scan is a form of diuresis renography. The right kidney curve is normal. After isotope injection, the ascending curve represents isotope uptake by the kidney. When frusemide is administered at 20 minutes, the curve falls sharply as the isotope is cleared into the lower urinary tract.

The left kidney is abnormal. Following frusemide administration, it fails to clear the isotope owing to the presence of a pelviureteric junction obstruction.

Notes

• Pelviureteric junction obstruction is more common in boys.
• An important cause of hydronephrosis, it may be detected on ante-natal ultrasonographic examination or present with loin pain and/or a loin mass. Some cases are asymptomatic.
• Complications include haematuria, urinary tract infection and hypertension.
• The treatment is pyeloplasty. If renal function is severely impaired drainage via a nephrostomy is indicated.
• Following a pyeloplasty the renogram curve should return to normal.

Gough DCS. The dilated urinary system. In: Postlethwaite RJ, ed. *Clinical Paediatric Nephrology.* 2nd ed. Oxford: Butterworth–Heinemann, 1994: 345–57.

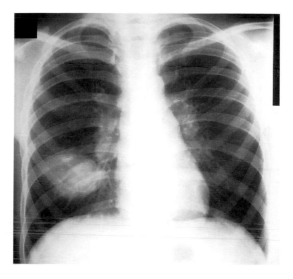

Question

This child has cystic fibrosis.

What is the additional diagnosis?

CASE 5.19

Answers

Allergic bronchopulmonary aspergillosis

Aspergillosis
Aspergilloma

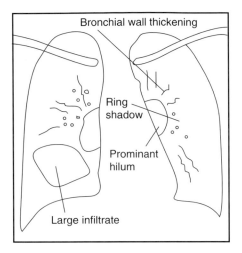

Picture description

There are changes compatible with cystic fibrosis: prominent hilum, ring shadows and bronchial wall thickening. The right lung field is overinflated and the right hilum enlarged. A large solid opacity is present within the right lower zone.

Notes

- *Aspergillus* is a mould that grows on decaying vegetable matter, liberating its spores into the air.
- The obstruction and impaired clearance of the airway in cystic fibrosis (CF) encourages colonization by *Aspergillus*.
- The main species causing lung problems is *Aspergillus fumigatus*. Three conditions are recognized: aspergilloma, allergic bronchopulmonary aspergillosis and invasive aspergillosis.
- **Aspergillomas** may form following the colonization of a cavity (e.g. secondary to tuberculosis). A rounded mass with surrounding air is seen on the radiograph. Aspergillomas are very uncommon in CF.
- In CF, **allergic bronchopulmonary aspergillosis** (ABPA) is the main condition caused by *Aspergillus*:
  - (i) The diagnosis should be considered when an infiltrate fails to clear with appropriate antibiotic therapy.

230

(ii) Diagnostic criteria include reversible bronchoconstriction, blood eosinophilia, raised IgE level, positive serum precipitins and specific IgE to *A. fumigatus.*

(iii) Single or multiple infiltrates are seen on chest radiography. They appear solid but may be cavitated on computed tomography.

(iv) Oral steroids are used to relieve symptoms and to prevent residual bronchiectasis.

Hiller EJ. Pathogenesis and management of aspergillosis in cystic fibrosis. *Archives of Disease in Childhood* 1990; **65**: 397–8.

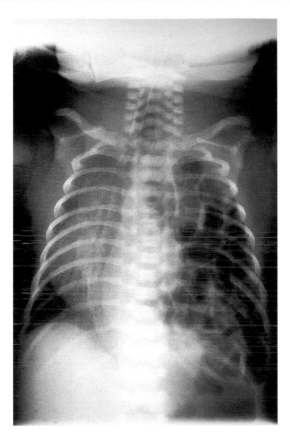

Question

This is a chest radiograph of a newborn baby.

What is the diagnosis?

Answers

Left-sided congenital diaphragmatic hernia
Left-sided congenital diaphragmatic hernia with mediastinal shift to the right

Congenital diaphragmatic hernia
Diaphragmatic hernia

Cystic adenomatoid malformation of the lung

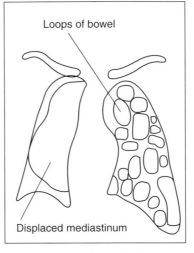

Picture description

The infant is intubated. There are multiple loops of bowel within the left hemithorax with mediastinal displacement to the right side.

Notes

- A congenital diaphragmatic hernia results when the pleuroperitoneal folds fail to fuse with the septum transversum in the seventh week of embryonic life.
- The incidence is 1 in 2000. Eighty-five per cent are left-sided.
- Antenatal diagnosis may be difficult. On ultrasonographic examination, the differential diagnosis is cystic adenomatoid malformation of the lung and mediastinal cystic teratoma.
- Abdominal organs herniate into the thoracic cavity, compressing the lungs, resulting in pulmonary hypoplasia.
- One-third have other congenital abnormalities, such as congenital heart disease.

- Labour ward management: avoid resuscitation with a bag and mask (this can make the situation worse), secure airway by endotracheal intubation, deflate gut with a nasogastric tube on free drainage, provide ventilatory support.
- Mortality is reduced by stabilizing before operation. Infants need to be sedated and paralysed.
- The defect is repaired with a primary closure or a GORE-TEX (polytetrafluoroethylene) patch if the defect is large.
- The prognosis is poor with severe hypoxia not responding to treatment.

Examination 6

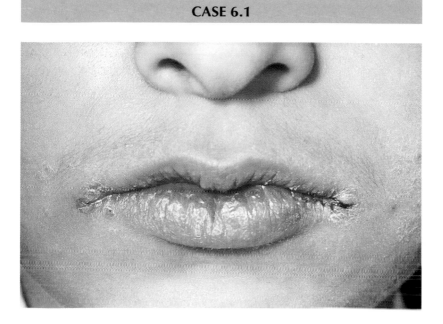

Question

This patient has finger clubbing.

What is the underlying diagnosis?

Answers

Crohn's disease

Inflammatory bowel disease

Picture description

The lips are inflamed (cheilitis) and the skin at the corners of the mouth is cracked.

Notes

- Crohn's disease has a prevalence of 30–100 per 100000.
- Presenting features include abdominal pain, diarrhoea, anorexia, weight loss, rectal bleeding and poor growth.
- Eighty per cent of cases have disease involving the ileum with or without colonic involvement. Up to 20% have isolated colonic disease.
- Extraintestinal manifestations include arthritis, erythema nodosum, pyoderma gangrenosum and uveitis.
- Endoscopic findings include focal or segmental inflammation, aphthous ulceration and cobblestoning.
- Complications include obstruction, fistulae, abscesses, perianal disease and vitamin B_{12} deficiency.
- Drug therapy does not alter the long-term course of Crohn's disease (in contrast to ulcerative colitis). Treatment is aimed at controlling symptoms.
- Oral prednisolone induces remission in 70% of patients. Sulphasalazine is used as an adjunct to prednisolone for colonic disease. Metronidazole is the drug of choice for perianal disease.
- Surgical intervention is indicated for bowel perforation or obstruction, intractable bleeding and fistula drainage.

Hofley PM, Piccoli DA. Inflammatory bowel disease in children. *Medical Clinics of North America* 1994; **78**: 1281–302.

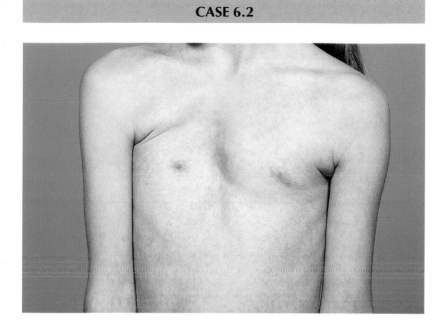

Question

This 10 year old girl had an abnormal left hand.

What is the most likely diagnosis?

Answers

Poland syndrome

Absent pectoralis major muscle
Muscle wasting

Picture description

The right pectoralis major muscle is absent.

Notes

- Poland syndrome is a congenital absence of the pectoralis major muscle with ipsilateral deformity of the upper limb.
- Incidence 1 in 25 000 live births. Most cases are sporadic.
- There is a variable degree of hypoplasia of the breast, subcutaneous tissue, muscle and ribs.
- Other associated anomalies include scoliosis, Sprengel's deformity, dextrocardia, pectus excavatum and renal hypoplasia.
- Chest wall reconstruction can be performed with a latissimus dorsi muscle flap and an artificial breast implant.

Marks MW, Argenta LC, Izenburg PH, Mes LGB. Management of the chest-wall deformity in male patients with Poland's syndrome. *Plastic and Reconstructive Surgery* 1991; **87**: 674–8.

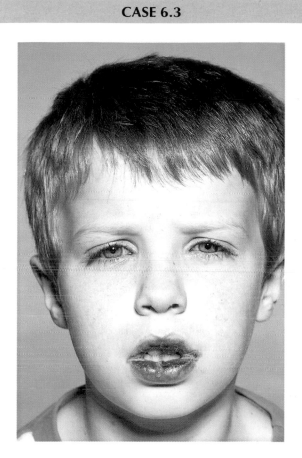

Question

What is this diagnosis?

Answer

Stevens–Johnson syndrome

Picture description

Severe conjunctivitis and oral stomatitis.

Notes

- Stevens–Johnson syndrome is a serious systemic form of erythema multiforme in which the skin and at least two mucous membranes are involved.
- The mucosa of the conjunctivae, lips, genitalia, nose and mouth may become eroded.
- Patients are at risk of fluid loss, anaemia and infection.
- The mortality rate can be as high as 10%, particularly in cases with pulmonary lesions.
- Treatment is supportive with close attention to fluid and electrolyte replacement. Intensive care may be required.
- Regular ophthalmological assessment is important.
- The use of systemic steroids is controversial.

Eichenfield LF, Honig PJ. Blistering disorders in childhood. *Pediatric Clinics of North America* 1991; **38**: 959–76.

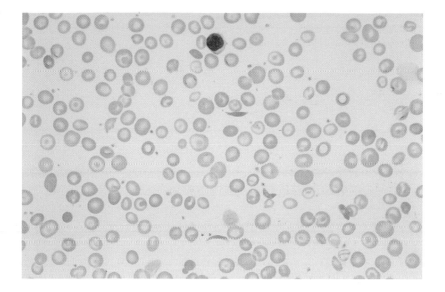

Questions

(a) List three abnormal cells on this blood film.

(b) What is the most likely diagnosis?

Answers

(a) Target cells
     Sickle cells
     Spherocytes
     Reticulocytes

(b) Sickle cell disease

Picture description

In addition to the above, the red blood cells demonstrate hypochromia, poikilocytosis (variation in cell shape), anisocytosis (variation in cell size) and polychromasia (blue colour change). A spherocyte can be seen in the lower left-hand corner of the slide.

Notes

- Sickle cell disease is common in African, Afro-Caribbean, Middle Eastern and Indian people. The importantly sickling genotypes are homozygous sickle cell (SS) and sickle cell haemoglobin C (SC).
- Sickle haemoglobin (HbS) results from the substitution of valine for glutamic acid on the β-globulin chain. Deoxygenated HbS causes sickling of the red blood cell and the blockage of blood flow in the microcirculation.
- In SS disease the red cells contain more than 80% HbS, the remainder being fetal haemoglobin.
- Antenatal diagnosis is possible using samples obtained from chorionic villus sampling or amniocentesis.
- A chronic haemolytic anaemia is characteristic (Hb level 6–9 g/dl). Pigment gallstones may form.
- Dactylitis is pathognomonic of SS disease, occurring within the first 4 months of life.
- The acute chest syndrome (pleuritic pain, dyspnoea, lung consolidation) is the commonest cause of mortality after 2 years of age.
- Acute splenic sequestration presents with anaemia and shock secondary to rapid enlargement of the spleen. Blood transfusion is essential.
- Pneumococcal vaccination and prophylactic penicillin V are important measures to prevent pneumococcal septicaemia.
- Bone marrow transplantation is curative but carries the risk of graft failure.
- Hydroxyurea increases HbF production and reduces the incidence of severe crises.

Serjeant GR. Recent advances in sickle cell disease. In: David TJ, ed. *Recent Advances in Paediatrics*, Vol. 12. Edinburgh: Churchill Livingstone, 1994: 141–54.

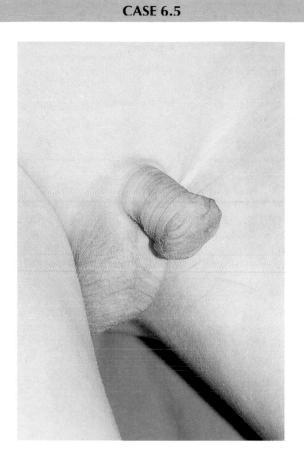

Questions

(a) What is the physical abnormality?

(b) What is the underlying diagnosis?

Answers

(a)   Hooded foreskin

(b)   Hypospadias

Notes

- Hypospadias is a common congenital defect occurring in 1 in 300 boys.
- It is defined by three anatomical anomalies of the penis:
    (i)   An abnormal ventral opening of the urethral meatus, which can be classified as glanular, coronal, mid-shaft or penoscrotal.
    (ii) An abnormal curvature of the penis (chordee).
    (iii) A hooded foreskin due to a ventral deficiency of skin.
- Surgical reconstruction is delayed until the second or third year of life.
- Post-operative complications include fistula and urethral stenosis.

Mouriquand PDE, Persad R, Sharma S. Hypospadias repair: current principles and procedures. *British Journal of Urology* 1995; **76** (Suppl 3): 9–22.

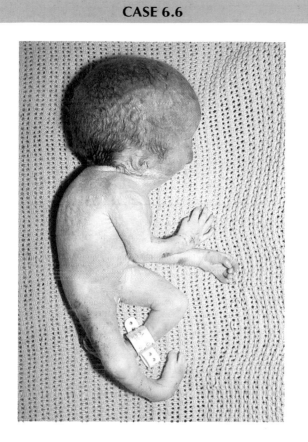

Question

What is the diagnosis?

Answers

Camptomelic dystrophy

Dwarfism

Picture description

This child was stillborn. The dysmorphic features are a prominent forehead, micrognathia, a deformed pinna, short bowed legs and talipes equinovarus.

Notes

- Camptomelic dysplasia is characterized by short stature, short limbs, and bowing of the long bones.
- The majority of cases are phenotypic females.
- Infants tend to be stillborn, or die during the neonatal period from respiratory complications.
- The diagnosis is confirmed on a skeletal survey (cloverleaf skull, mid-femur angulation, long bone bowing, hypoplastic scapulae).

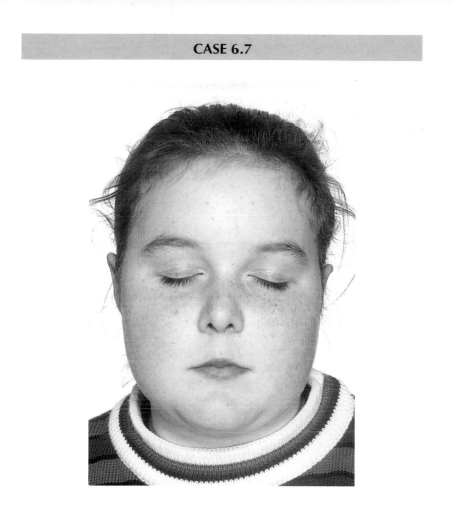

Question

This 12 year old girl presented to her general practitioner with difficulty climbing stairs at school.

(a) What is the most likely diagnosis?

(b) What is the most useful test to confirm your diagnosis ?

Answers

(a) Dermatomyositis

Connective tissue disease
Systemic lupus erythematosus

(b) Muscle biopsy

Serum muscle enzyme concentrations

Picture description

There is purple discolouration of the eyelids (heliotrope).

Notes

- Dermatomyositis is an inflammatory disease of muscle and skin. The cause is unknown.
- It can occur at any age. Girls are affected more commonly than boys.
- The childhood form differs from the adult form because it is not associated with occult malignancy.
- The rash is a symmetrical, scaly erythema of the face and extensor surfaces (knuckles, elbows, knees). It has a violaceous or heliotrope hue that is most prominent on the eyelids and nasal bridge.
- The essential diagnostic criteria are proximal muscle weakness, the characteristic rash, raised muscle enzyme levels, electromyographic evidence of an inflammatory myopathy, and chronic muscle inflammation on histology.
- The disease may present acutely, or insidiously with fatigue, fever, arthralgia and rash. Sun exposure is a precipitating factor.
- Treatment consists of physiotherapy and prednisolone. Methotrexate, cyclosporin and immunoglobulins have been used successfully.

Jones EM, Callen JP. Collagen vascular diseases of childhood. *Pediatric Clinics of North America* 1991; **38**: 1019–39.

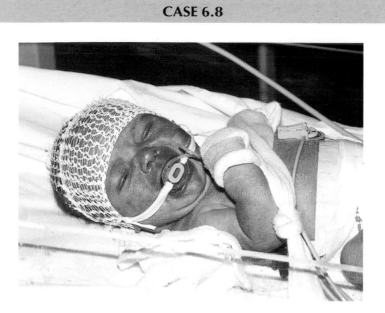

Question

What is the most likely diagnosis?

Answers

Bilateral choanal atresia

Choanal atresia

Picture description

The infant has an oropharyngeal airway *in situ.*

Notes

- Choanal atresia is the commonest form of nasal obstruction in the newborn. It results from a unilateral or bilateral, bony or membranous, obstruction in the posterior nares.
- The incidence is 1:60 000 births. Male to female ratio is 1:2.
- Bony atresia accounts for up to 90% of cases.
- Bilateral obstruction presents in the newborn period with respiratory distress. The inability to pass a firm nasogastric tube into the nasopharynx suggests the diagnosis.
- Unilateral obstruction may present early with feeding difficulties or later with a persistent nasal discharge.
- In 60% of cases, choanal atresia is associated with other congenital abnormalities (congenital heart defects, Treacher-Collins and CHARGE syndromes).
- The inability to pass a firm nasogastric tube into the nasopharynx suggests the diagnosis.
- Direct fibreoptic examination and high resolution computed tomography (CT) will confirm the diagnosis.
- Surgery is undertaken as soon as the infant is fit for general anaesthesia. Re-stenosis is a recognized complication.

Prescott CAJ. Nasal obstruction in infancy. *Archives of Disease in Childhood* 1995; **72**: 287–9

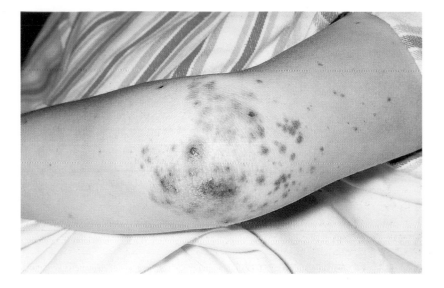

Question

This 9 year old boy presented with haematuria.

What is the most likely diagnosis?

Answers

Henoch–Schoenlein purpura

Idiopathic thrombocytopenic purpura
Meningococcal septicaemia

Acute post-streptococcal glomerulonephritis
Systemic lupus erythematosus
Connective tissue disease

Meningococcal meningitis

Picture description

The left elbow is swollen and covered by a purpuric rash with a small number of vesicles.

Notes

- Henoch–Schoenlein purpura (HSP) is a common vasculitis of unknown aetiology, often preceded by an upper respiratory tract infection.
- It commonly occurs between the ages 2 and 8 years, affecting more boys than girls.
- The characteristic purpuric rash involves the lower extremities and buttocks. Small vesicles and areas of desquamation may develop.
- Colicky abdominal pain is common, with melaena in 20% and intussusception in 5% of cases.
- Periarticular joint swelling is transient, commonly affecting the knees, ankles and elbows.
- All children with renal involvement have proteinuria and haematuria. Nephrotic syndrome, acute nephritis and progressive renal failure can occur.
- Antinuclear antibody and rheumatoid factor are negative. C3 levels are normal. The stools are positive for blood in 50% of patients.
- Management is conservative except in cases of severe abdominal pain and haemorrhage, when steroid therapy may be beneficial.

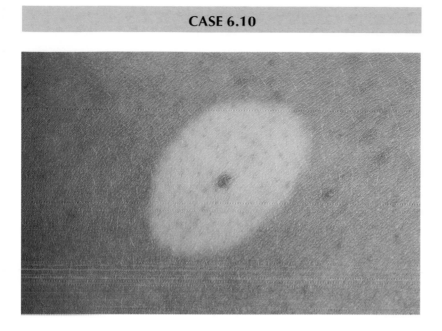

Questions

What is the diagnosis?

Answers

(a) Halo naevus

Vitiligo

Melanocytic naevus

Picture description

A central melanocytic naevus is surrounded by an area of depigmentation.

Notes

- Halo naevi occur primarily in children and young adults, most commonly on the back.
- The central naevus involutes over several months leaving a pale area which may take years to repigment.
- They are harmless and excision is not necessary.

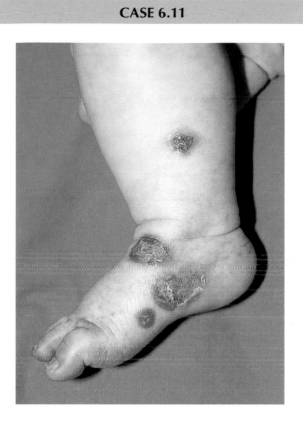

Question

What is the diagnosis?

Answers

Bullous impetigo
Impetigo

Staphylococcal scalded skin syndrome

Picture description

There are multiple ruptured bullae with superficial crusts on the dorsal surface of the right foot and lower leg.

Notes

- Impetigo is a local reaction between invading organisms and neutrophils.
- **Non-bullous** impetigo accounts for 70% of cases. Transient vesicles develop into exuding lesions with yellow crusts and surrounding erythema. The face and limbs are commonly affected.
- **Bullous** impetigo occurs mainly in infants and young children. The bullae rupture to leave superficial crusts. The face, buttocks, perineum and limbs are commonly affected.
- Infections are usually caused by *Staphylococcus aureus*. However, non-bullous impetigo can be caused by *Streptococcus pyogenes*.
- Treatment with antibiotics is superior to cleansing with antiseptic solutions.
- Complications are rare, but include osteomyelitis, septic arthritis and post-streptococcal glomerulonephritis.
- Staphylococcal infection can cause 'scalded skin syndrome' – widespread superficial shedding of the epidermis.

Questions

This 12 year old boy was confined to a wheelchair.

(a)   What is the abnormal feature of the eye?

(b)   What is the diagnosis?

Answers

(a) Bulbar conjunctival telangiectasia

   Telangiectasia

   Conjunctivitis
   Episcleritis

(b) Ataxia telangiectasia

   Conjunctivitis
   Reiter's disease

Picture description

Telangiectasia are present on the bulbar conjunctiva and skin surrounding the eye.

Notes

- Ataxia telangiectasia is characterized by ataxia, oculocutaneous abnormalities, endocrine abnormalities, chronic infections and immune deficiency.
- The gene is located on the long arm of chromosome 11 (11q23).
- Progressive cerebellar ataxia develops soon after the child begins to walk.
- Oculocutaneous telangiectasia develops at between 3 and 6 years of age.
- The majority of patients suffer from recurrent pulmonary infections.
- DNA repair mechanisms are defective and there is an increased sensitivity to ionizing radiation. The incidence of lymphoreticular neoplasia is increased.
- Fifty per cent have selective IgA deficiency. IgG_2 and IgE levels are often low.
- Alpha-fetoprotein levels are raised.

Buckley RH. Immunodeficiency. *Journal of the American Medical Association* 1992; **268**: 2797–806.

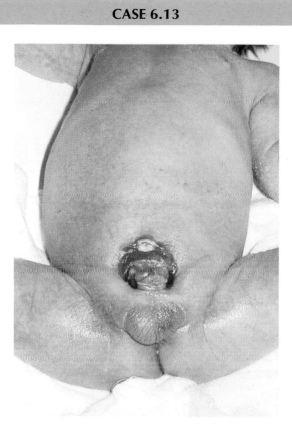

Question

What is the diagnosis?

Answer

Bladder exstrophy/ectopia vesicae with epispadias

Picture description

The bladder is everted on to the lower abdominal wall. An epispadias is present. A small scrotal sack suggests that the testes are undescended.

Notes

- Bladder exstrophy is due to the failure of development of the anterior abdominal wall and anterior bladder.
- Incidence 1 in 10000. It is more common in males.
- Antenatal ultrasonographic diagnosis is possible. Maternal serum and amniotic fluid alpha-fetoprotein levels are raised.
- The management aim is for complete urinary continence and preservation of the upper urinary tract.
- Primary bladder closure and pelvic osteotomy are commonly performed in the newborn period, with secondary bladder neck construction and epispadias repair during early childhood.
- Urinary diversion is necessary if the bladder is too small or fails to contract.

Stein R, Fisch M, Stockle M, Hohenfellner R. Urinary diversion in bladder exstrophy and incontinent epispadias: 25 years of experience. *Journal of Urology* 1995; **154**: 1177–81.

Question

What is the diagnosis?

Answers

Strawberry naevus
Capillary haemangioma

Picture description

There is a bright red, sharply demarcated, protuberant lesion on the trunk.

Notes

- Strawberry naevi may be present at birth, but usually appear within the first 2 months of life.
- Common sites are the face, scalp, back and anterior chest.
- Lesions may be solitary or multiple.
- Approximately 60% involute by 5 years, 95% by 9 years.
- Complications include ulceration, infection and haemorrhage.
- A lesion requires treatment only if it compromises a vital function such as vision.

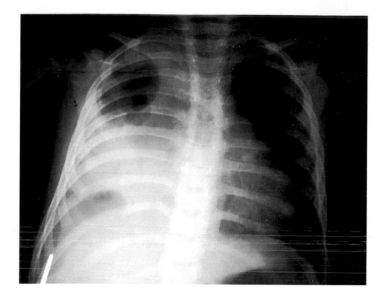

Question

Chest radiography was performed on this 1 year old child.

What is the most likely diagnosis?

Answers

Right-sided staphylococcal pneumonia

Right-sided empyema
Right-sided pleural effusion

Pneumonia
Lung abscess

Tuberculosis
Lung cyst
Pneumothorax

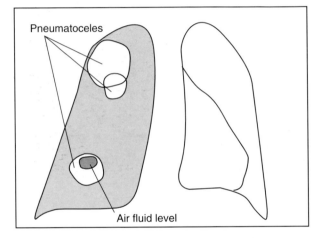

Picture description

There are multiple, spherical, air-containing lesions (pneumatocoeles) within the consolidated right hemithorax.

Notes

- Pneumatoceles are very rare, except in staphylococcal pneumonia.
- They usually appear 1 week after the onset of the infection.
- Resolution is complete following successful treatment of the pneumonia.

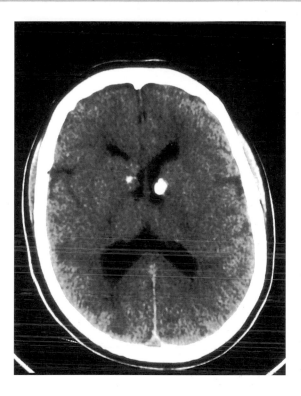

Question

This scan is from a 16 year old girl with learning difficulties.

What is the diagnosis?

Answer

Tuberous sclerosis

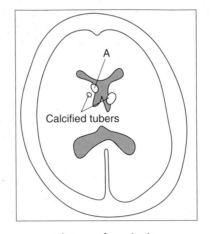

Picture description

There are multiple subependymal calcified tubers. The nodule (A), within the lateral wall of the right frontal horn, is enhanced with contrast and probably represents an astrocytoma.

Notes

- Tuberous sclerosis has an incidence of 1 in 6000.
- Two genes have been located: *TSC1* on chromosome 9q and *TSC2* on chromosome 16q.
- Inheritance is autosomal dominant; two-thirds of cases are new mutations.
- Clinical features:
    - seizures – infantile spasms, complex partial, myoclonic.
    - skin lesions – ash-leaf macules, forehead fibrous plaque, shagreen patch, periungal fibromas, facial angiofibromas.
    - cardiac rhabdomyomas (eighty per cent of children with cardiac rhabdomyomas have tuberous sclerosis).
    - renal disease – polycystic kidneys, angiomyolipomas.
    - subependymal calcified tubers (which may enlarge causing obstructive hydrocephalus) and giant cell astrocytomas.
    - behavioural disorders – autism, hyperactivity.
    - developmental delay.
- Over 50% of affected patients have normal intelligence.

Webb DW, Osborne JP. Tuberous sclerosis. *Archives of Disease in Childhood* 1995; **72**: 471–4.

Questions

This child has chronic renal failure.

(a) Describe the bony abnormality.

(b) What is the most likely underlying cause for this finding?

Answers

(a) Subperiosteal erosions

(b) Secondary hyperparathyroidism

Metabolic bone disease secondary to chronic renal failure
Renal osteodystrophy

Rickets

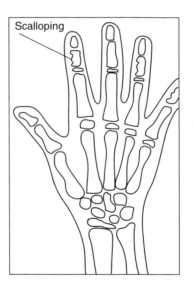

Picture description

The bone on the radial side of the middle phalanges is irregularly scalloped.

Notes

- Renal osteodystrophy occurs in up to 80% of children with chronic renal failure.
- Declining renal function leads to hyperphosphataemia and reduced 1,25-dihydroxy vitamin D production. As a consequence bone mineralization is impaired and intestinal calcium absorption reduced. The fall in plasma ionized calcium concentration stimulates the parathyroid gland, resulting in secondary hyperparathyroidism.
- Clinical features of renal osteodystrophy include bone pain, muscle weakness and pathological fractures.

- Radiological features include widening, cupping and fraying of the epiphysis.
- Renal bone disease is managed with a low phosphate diet, calcium carbonate (as a phosphate binder), and 1α-hydroxycholecalciferol supplements.

Mughal Z. Disorders of mineral metabolism as a presenting feature of renal disease. In: Postlethwaite RJ, ed. *Clinical Paediatric Nephrology*. 2nd edition. Oxford: Butterworth Heinemann, 1994: 48–58.

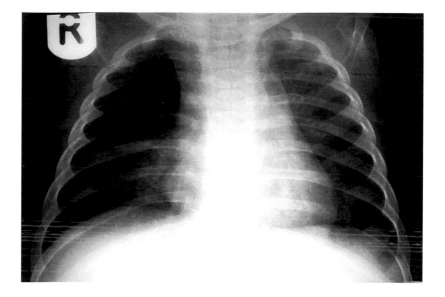

Question

This 9 month old boy had been tachypnoeic since birth.

What is the most likely diagnosis?

Answers

Right upper lobe congenital lobar emphysema
Right-sided congenital lung cyst

Congenital lobar emphysema
Congenital lung cyst

Congenital adenomatoid malformation
Diaphragmatic hernia
Foreign body inhalation

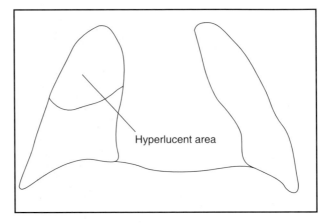

Hyperlucent area

Picture description

The right upper lobe is hyperinflated and hyperlucent.
A diagnosis of pneumothorax is unlikely as lung markings are present in
the right lower zone.

Notes

- Congenital lobar emphysema frequently affects the left upper lobe.
- In many cases the condition is attributed to defective bronchial
  cartilage.
- Up to 30% of cases have an associated cardiac defect.
- Clinical features: respiratory distress, hyperinflation, reduced breath
  sounds, expiratory wheeze on the affected side.
- Mildly symptomatic infants are treated conservatively.
- Lobectomy is indicated in the presence of severe respiratory distress.

Questions

This preterm infant rapidly developed severe respiratory distress.

What is the underlying cause for this deterioration?

Answer

Pneumoperitoneum

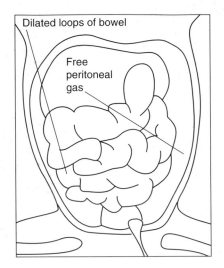

Picture description

The bowel is dilated. There is a large amount of free gas within the peritoneum.

Notes

- A pneumoperitoneum may result from perforation of the gut or from air dissecting through the diaphragmatic foramina into the peritoneum in ventilated babies.
- A lateral decubitus radiograph may be required to diagnose small leaks.
- Predisposing conditions: necrotizing enterocolitis, Hirschprung's disease, meconium ileus and corticosteroid therapy.
- Drainage of the peritoneum (by needle aspiration or by inserting a drain) is necessary only in the presence of severe respiratory or circulatory embarrassment.

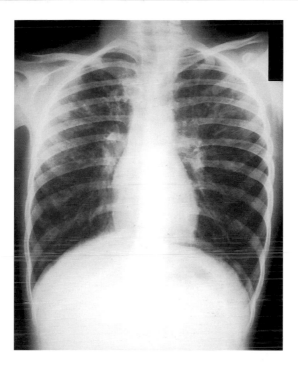

Questions

(a) List three abnormalities on this chest radiograph.

(b) What is the most likely diagnosis?

Answers

(a) Hyperinflation
Bronchial thickening
Ring shadows
Bilateral upper lobe nodular infiltrates
Prominent hilar lymph nodes

(b) Cystic fibrosis

Pneumonia
Aspiration

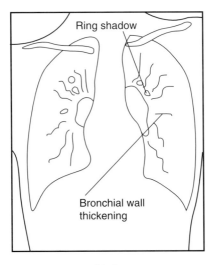

Ring shadow

Bronchial wall thickening

Notes

- Cystic fibrosis is an autosomal recessive disorder with an incidence of 1 in 2500 Caucasian live births.
- The gene is located on the long arm of chromosome 7. One in 25 of the population are carriers.
- More than 300 mutations have been identified. Up to 75% of children in the UK have the $\Delta F508$ mutation.
- Production of an abnormal cystic fibrosis transmembrane conductance regulator (CFTR) protein leads to defective chloride ion transport.
- Antenatal diagnosis is possible using chorionic villus biopsy samples.
- Presenting features: chest infection (55%), malabsorption (30%) meconium ileus (15%).
- Neonatal programmes screen for raised serum immunoreactive trypsin (IRT) levels.

- The diagnosis is confirmed by two positive sweat tests: sodium >70 mmol/kg, weight of sweat >100 mg.
- The median age of survival is 25 years of age.
- Gene replacement therapy into the respiratory tract has been attempted using adenovirus and liposomal vectors.

Caplen N *et al.* Liposome-mediated CFTR gene transfer to the nasal epithelium of patients with cystic fibrosis. *Nature Medicine* 1995; 1: 39–46.

Index

Numbers in *italics* refer to illustrations